# The New Menopause Diet Cookbook

## An Ultimate Guide to Delicious Recipes and Easy Hormonal Change

Dr Olivia Tastewell

# Copyright © 2024 by Dr Olivia Tastewell



*For permission requests, write to the author at droliviatastewell@gmail.com*
*Kindly scan the bar code below to reach out to the author and have access to more of our books.*

# TABLE OF CONTENTS

# INTRODUCTION

IMAGINE YOU ARE MRS HUDSON, a woman in her late forties who is going through menopause. You have been feeling the effects of this life-changing transition for a while now, and you are not happy about it. You are tired of the hot flashes, the mood swings, the weight gain, the insomnia, and the other symptoms that make you feel miserable. You are frustrated by the lack of information and support you get from your doctor, your family, and your friends. You are confused by the conflicting advice and opinions you hear from the media, the internet, and the books you read. You are disappointed by the solutions and remedies you try, from hormone replacement therapy to herbal supplements that either don't work or have unpleasant side effects.

 You are desperate for a way to cope with the changes and challenges that menopause brings, and to improve your health and well-being.

You are not alone. Millions of women around the world are going through the same thing as you, and they are looking for the same thing as you: a simple and effective way to manage their hormonal changes and improve their quality of life. A way that is natural, safe, and enjoyable. A way that involves one of the most basic and essential aspects of life: food.

That's where this book comes in. This book is the result of my own personal journey with menopause and the new menopause diet, a revolutionary approach that changed my life for the better, and that can change yours too. In this book, I will share with you my story and experience, and show you how you can benefit from the new menopause diet too. I will teach you everything you need to know about menopause and hormonal change, and how to manage them with nutrition and diet. I will also give you over 100 delicious and nutritious recipes that follow the new menopause diet principles and guidelines, as well as a sample meal plan, a shopping list, and some tips and tricks on how to follow the diet easily and effectively.

Finally, I will also share with you some success stories and testimonials from real women who have tried and benefited from the new menopause diet, as well as some advice and guidance on how to maintain and sustain the diet in the long term,

and how to cope with potential challenges and setbacks. This book is more than just a cookbook. It's a lifestyle guide that will show you how to enjoy delicious food and manage hormonal change with ease and confidence. It's a book that will help you achieve your health and wellness goals, and transform your life for the better. It's a book that will make you love your menopause journey, and embrace this new phase of your life.

So, are you ready to go on this adventure with me? Are you ready to discover the secrets of the new menopause diet, and how to create tasty recipes that support your hormones and improve your health? Are you ready to eat well and feel great during menopause, and beyond? If you are, then let's get started. Grab your apron, your knife, and your cutting board, and let's head to the kitchen. The new menopause diet cookbook awaits you.

# Chapter 1: Understanding Menopause and Hormonal Change

If you are reading this book, chances are you are either going through menopause or perimenopause, or you are curious about what to expect when you do. Either way, you probably have a lot of questions and concerns about this life stage, and how it affects your body and mind. You may also have some myths and misconceptions about menopause, and some fears and anxieties about the changes and challenges it brings. Don't worry, you are not alone. Menopause is a natural and inevitable part of biological ageing for women, and it affects millions of women around the world. It is also a unique and personal experience for each woman, and it can have a significant impact on your physical, emotional, mental, and social well-being. That's why it is important to understand what menopause is, and how it affects your body and mind. In this chapter, we will explain what menopause is, and how it affects your hormones, which are the chemical messengers that regulate many functions and processes in your body.

We will also discuss the common symptoms and challenges of menopause, such as hot flashes, mood swings, weight gain, insomnia, and more. We will also provide some tips and suggestions on how to cope with them, and how to improve your health and happiness during this transition.

By the end of this chapter, you will have a better understanding of menopause and hormonal change, and you will be more prepared and confident to face this new phase of your life. You will also be ready to learn more about the new menopause diet, a revolutionary approach that will help you manage your hormonal changes and enjoy your food, which we will introduce in the next chapter.

So, let's get started. Grab a cup of tea, a pen, and a notebook, and let's dive into the fascinating world of menopause and hormonal change.

# What is menopause and how does it affect your body and mind?

Menopause is the point in time when a woman's ovaries stop producing eggs and release fewer female hormones, mainly estrogen and progesterone. This means that a woman can no longer get pregnant naturally, and her menstrual periods stop permanently. Menopause is considered to have occurred after 12 consecutive months without menstruation, for which there is no other obvious physiological or pathological cause, and in the absence of clinical intervention.

The average age of natural menopause is around 51 years, but it can vary from woman to woman, depending on various factors, such as genetics, lifestyle, health conditions, and environmental exposures. Some women may experience menopause earlier (before 40 years of age), which is called premature menopause, or later (after 55 years of age), which is called late menopause. Some women may also experience menopause as a result of surgical or medical procedures that affect their ovaries, such as hysterectomy (removal of the uterus), oophorectomy (ovarian removal), chemotherapy, or radiation treatment for cancer.

Menopause is not a sudden event, but a gradual process that can take several years. The period leading up to menopause, when a woman's ovaries start to produce fewer eggs and hormones, and her menstrual cycle becomes irregular, is called perimenopause. Perimenopause can start as early as the late 30s or as late as the early 50s, and it can last from a few months to several years. The period after menopause, when a woman's hormone levels have stabilized at a low level, is called postmenopause.

Menopause affects your body and mind in many ways, because hormones play a vital role in regulating many functions and processes in your body, such as reproduction, metabolism, growth, development, mood, cognition, and more. When your hormone levels change during menopause, you may experience various physical, emotional, mental, and social changes, which can affect your health and well-being.

Some of these changes are normal and expected, and some of them are temporary and reversible. Some of these changes may not bother you at all, and some of them may be mild and manageable. However, some of these changes may be severe and distressing, and may require medical attention and treatment.

In the next section, we will discuss some of the most common symptoms and challenges of menopause, and how to cope with them.

# Symptoms and Challenges of Menopause

The symptoms and challenges of menopause vary from woman to woman, depending on various factors, such as genetics, lifestyle, health conditions, and environmental exposures. Some women may have few or no symptoms, while others may have many and severe symptoms. Some women may have symptoms that start before menopause, and some may have symptoms that continue after menopause. Some women may have symptoms that come and go, and some may have symptoms that persist.

The most common symptoms and challenges of menopause are:

- Hot flashes and night sweats: These are sudden sensations of heat that spread over the face, neck, chest, and sometimes the whole body, accompanied by sweating, flushing, and palpitations.

They can last from a few seconds to several minutes, and can occur several times a day or night. They can cause discomfort, embarrassment, sleep disturbance, and fatigue. They are caused by changes in the brain's temperature regulation, which are influenced by estrogen levels. They usually start during perimenopause, and can last for a few months to several years. They tend to be more frequent and intense in women who smoke, are overweight, or have a history of hot flashes in their family.

- Vaginal dryness and discomfort: This is the thinning, drying, and inflammation of the vaginal lining, which can cause itching, burning, irritation, and pain during sexual intercourse. It can also increase the risk of vaginal infections and urinary tract infections. It is caused by the decrease in estrogen levels, which affects the production of natural lubrication and the elasticity of the vaginal tissue.

It usually starts during perimenopause, and can last indefinitely. It tends to be more severe in women who smoke, have diabetes, or have a history of vaginal dryness in their family.

- Mood changes: These are fluctuations in mood, such as feeling sad, anxious, irritable, angry, or stressed. They can also include depression, which is a persistent and severe low mood that interferes with daily functioning. They are caused by a combination of factors, such as hormonal changes, life stressors, sleep problems, physical symptoms, and personal and social changes. They usually start during perimenopause, and can last for a few months to several years. They tend to be more common and intense in women who have a history of mood disorders, such as premenstrual syndrome (PMS), postpartum depression, or bipolar disorder.

- Weight gain and changes in body shape:These are increases in body weight and fat, especially around the abdomen, hips, and thighs. They can also include changes in muscle mass and bone density, which can affect strength, posture, and balance.

They are caused by a combination of factors, such as hormonal changes, ageing, metabolism, diet, physical activity, and genetics. They usually start during perimenopause, and can last indefinitely.

They tend to be more pronounced in women who are sedentary, eat poorly, or have a history of weight problems in their family.

- Insomnia and sleep problems: These are difficulties in falling asleep, staying asleep, or getting enough quality sleep. They can also include sleep apnea, which is a condition where breathing stops and starts repeatedly during sleep. They can cause daytime fatigue, impaired concentration, memory loss, and mood changes. They are caused by a combination of factors, such as hormonal changes, hot flashes, night sweats, stress, anxiety, depression, and other medical conditions. They usually start during perimenopause, and can last for a few months to several years. They tend to be more frequent and severe in women who smoke, drink alcohol, or have a history of sleep problems in their family.

These are some of the most common symptoms and challenges of menopause, but they are not the only ones. Some women may also experience other symptoms and challenges, such as:

- Changes in sexual function and desire: These are changes in the ability and interest to have sexual activity, such as having less or more desire, arousal, orgasm, or satisfaction. They can also include changes in sexual identity and orientation, such as feeling more or less feminine, masculine, or bisexual. They are caused by a combination of factors, such as hormonal changes, vaginal dryness, discomfort, pain, mood changes, stress, relationship issues, and self-image. They usually start during perimenopause, and can last indefinitely. They tend to vary widely from woman to woman, and from time to time.

- Changes in memory and cognition: These are changes in the ability to think, learn, remember, and process information, such as having difficulty concentrating, recalling names, words, or numbers, or multitasking.

They can also include changes in creativity, intuition, and wisdom, such as having more or less insight, inspiration, or innovation. They are caused by a combination of factors, such as hormonal changes, ageing, sleep problems, mood changes, stress, and other medical conditions. They usually start during perimenopause, and can last for a few months to several years. They tend to be mild and temporary, and do not affect daily functioning or intelligence.

- Changes in skin, hair, and nails: These are changes in the appearance and texture of the skin, hair, and nails, such as having more or less dryness, oiliness, wrinkles, sagging, spots, or hair loss. They can also include changes in sensitivity and sensation, such as having more or less itching.

## Role of Hormones in Menopause

Hormones are chemical messengers that travel through your bloodstream and affect various organs and tissues in your body.

They regulate many functions and processes, such as reproduction, metabolism, growth, development, mood, cognition, and more.

During menopause, your ovaries stop producing eggs and release fewer female hormones, mainly estrogen and progesterone. These hormones play a vital role in controlling your menstrual cycle, preparing your body for pregnancy, and maintaining your bone and cardiovascular health.

As your hormone levels decline, you may experience various changes in your body and mind, such as:

- Changes in your menstrual cycle: Your periods may become irregular, lighter, heavier, shorter, or longer, until they eventually stop.
- Changes in your reproductive system: Your vagina may become thinner, drier, and less elastic, causing discomfort, pain, or infections. Your uterus may shrink, and your pelvic floor muscles may weaken, leading to urinary incontinence or prolapse. Your breasts may lose firmness and fullness, and your nipples may become less sensitive.
- Changes in your bones and muscles: Your bones may lose density and strength, increasing your risk of fractures and osteoporosis.

Your muscles may lose mass and tone, affecting your strength, posture, and balance.

- Changes in your metabolism and weight: Your metabolism may slow down, and your body may store more fat, especially around your abdomen, hips, and thighs. You may gain weight or find it harder to lose weight.

- Changes in your cardiovascular system: Your blood pressure may rise, and your cholesterol and triglyceride levels may change, increasing your risk of heart disease and stroke. Your blood vessels may become less elastic and more prone to damage, affecting your blood flow and circulation.

- Changes in your skin, hair, and nails: Your skin may become thinner, drier, and more wrinkled, and may lose elasticity and collagen. Your hair may become thinner, coarser, and more brittle, and may fall out more easily. Your nails may become weaker, softer, and more prone to splitting and breaking.

- Changes in your nervous system and brain: Your brain may shrink slightly, and your nerve cells may become less efficient, affecting your memory, concentration, learning, and problem-solving. Your mood may fluctuate, and you may experience depression, anxiety, irritability, anger, or stress. Your sleep quality may deteriorate, and you may have insomnia, nightmares, or sleep apnea. Your senses may change, and you may have headaches, dizziness, or tinnitus.

- Changes in your immune system and inflammation: Your immune system may become weaker, and you may be more susceptible to infections, allergies, and autoimmune diseases. Your inflammation levels may increase, and you may have more pain, swelling, or stiffness in your joints, muscles, or tissues.

These changes can have a significant impact on your health and well-being, and may affect your quality of life, self-esteem, and relationships. However, not all women experience the same changes, and not all changes are negative or permanent.

Some changes may be mild and manageable, and some may even be positive or beneficial.

For example, some women may feel more confident, liberated, or empowered after menopause, and may enjoy their sexuality, creativity, or wisdom more. Some women may also have fewer or no symptoms, and may adapt well to the changes.

The way you experience menopause depends on various factors, such as your genetics, lifestyle, health conditions, and environmental exposures. It also depends on how you perceive and cope with the changes, and what kind of support and treatment you receive. That's why it is important to understand the role of hormones in menopause, and how they influence your health and well-being. By knowing what to expect and what to do, you can take charge of your menopause journey, and make it a positive and rewarding experience.

# Nutrition and Hormonal Balance for Improved Quality of Life

Nutrition and diet are essential for your health and well-being at any stage of life, but especially during menopause. What you eat and drink can have a significant effect on your hormonal changes, and on your physical, emotional, mental, and social well-being.

Eating a healthy, balanced, and varied diet can help you:

- Reduce the severity and frequency of menopausal symptoms, such as hot flashes, night sweats, vaginal dryness, mood swings, insomnia, and weight gain.
- Prevent or manage health risks and complications associated with menopause, such as osteoporosis, heart disease, stroke, diabetes, and cancer.
- Maintain or improve your body weight, shape, and composition, and prevent or treat obesity and metabolic syndrome.

- Support or enhance your bone and muscle health, and prevent or treat fractures, falls, and sarcopenia.
- Protect or boost your cardiovascular health, and prevent or treat hypertension, dyslipidemia, and atherosclerosis.
- Preserve or restore your skin, hair, and nail health, and prevent or treat dryness, wrinkles, sagging, hair loss, and nail damage.
- Improve or optimize your brain and nervous system health, and prevent or treat cognitive decline, dementia, depression, anxiety, and sleep problems.
- Strengthen or modulate your immune system and inflammation, and prevent or treat infections, allergies, and autoimmune diseases.
- Increase or balance your energy levels, and prevent or treat fatigue, weakness, or exhaustion.
- Regulate or stabilize your mood and emotions, and prevent or treat irritability, anger, stress, or sadness.
- Enhance or maintain your sexual function and desire, and prevent or treat discomfort, pain, or infections.

- Promote or sustain your overall health and well-being, and improve your quality of life, self-esteem, and relationships.

To achieve these benefits, you need to eat a diet that meets your nutritional needs and preferences, and that supports your hormonal balance and health. A good diet for menopause should include:

- Plenty of fruits, vegetables, and whole grains, especially those that are rich in fiber, antioxidants, phytoestrogens, and other beneficial compounds. These foods can help lower your cholesterol, blood pressure, and inflammation, and may also help reduce hot flashes and vaginal dryness.

  Aim for at least five portions of fruits and vegetables, and three portions of whole grains per day.

- Adequate amounts of protein, especially from lean sources, such as fish, poultry, eggs, dairy, beans, nuts, and seeds. Protein can help you feel full and satisfied, and can also help you maintain or build your muscle mass and strength.

  Aim for at least 0.8 grams of protein per kilogram of body weight per day, and include protein in every meal and snack.

- Moderate amounts of healthy fats, especially from sources that are high in omega-3 fatty acids, such as oily fish, flaxseeds, chia seeds, walnuts, and olive oil. Healthy fats can help lower your cholesterol, blood pressure, and inflammation, and may also help improve your mood, cognition, and skin health. Aim for at least two portions of oily fish per week, and use olive oil for cooking and dressing.

- Sufficient amounts of calcium and vitamin D, which are essential for your bone health and prevention of osteoporosis. Calcium can be found in dairy products, fortified plant milks, green leafy vegetables, tofu, almonds, and sesame seeds. Vitamin D can be made by your skin when exposed to sunlight, but you may also need to get it from food sources, such as oily fish, eggs, mushrooms, and fortified foods, or from supplements. Aim for at least 700 milligrams of calcium and 10 micrograms of vitamin D per day.

- Limited amounts of salt, sugar, and alcohol, which can have negative effects on your health and well-being. Salt raises blood pressure and raises the risk of heart disease and stroke. Sugar can increase your blood glucose and insulin levels, and contributes to weight gain and diabetes. Alcohol can interfere with your sleep quality, mood, and cognition, and increase your risk of breast cancer and osteoporosis. Aim for no more than 6 grams of salt, 30 grams of sugar, and 14 units of alcohol per week.

In addition to eating a healthy diet, you may also benefit from taking some supplements, such as:

- Multivitamins and minerals, which can help fill any gaps in your diet and provide you with the essential nutrients you need for your health and well-being. Look for a supplement that is specially formulated for women in menopause, and that contains the recommended amounts of vitamins and minerals for your age and stage of life.

- Phytoestrogens, which are plant compounds that have a similar structure and effect to estrogen.
They can help balance your hormones and reduce some of the symptoms of menopause, such as hot flashes, night sweats, and vaginal dryness. They can be found in foods such as soy, flaxseeds, lentils, chickpeas, and red clover, or in supplements such as isoflavones, lignans, or black cohosh. However, the safety and efficacy of phytoestrogens are not well established, and they may interact with some medications or health conditions, so consult your doctor before taking them.
- Probiotics, which are beneficial bacteria that live in your gut and help with your digestion, immunity, and metabolism. They can help improve your gut health and function, and may also help with your weight, mood, and cognition. They can be found in foods such as yogurt, kefir, sauerkraut, kimchi, and kombucha, or in supplements such as lactobacillus, bifidobacterium, or saccharomyces.

Nutrition and diet are important for your health and well-being during menopause, but they are not the only factors that matter. You also need to consider other aspects of your lifestyle, such as physical activity, stress management, sleep hygiene, and social support. These factors can also affect your hormonal changes and your quality of life, and they can also be influenced by your nutrition and diet. That's why, in the next chapter, we will introduce you to the concept and principles of the new menopause diet, a revolutionary approach that will help you balance your hormones and enjoy your food, while also taking into account your lifestyle and well-being. The new menopause diet is more than just a diet, it's a way of living and loving your menopause journey. Stay tuned.

# Chapter 2: The New Menopause Diet Basics

In the previous chapter, we learned about menopause and hormonal change, and how they affect your body and mind. We also learned about the importance of nutrition and diet in managing your hormonal changes and improving your quality of life.

In this chapter, we will introduce you to the new menopause diet, a revolutionary approach that will help you balance your hormones and enjoy your food, while also taking into account your lifestyle and well-being. The new menopause diet is more than just a diet, it's a way of living and loving your menopause journey. The new menopause diet is based on the latest scientific research and evidence, as well as the wisdom and experience of women who have successfully followed it. It is designed to suit your individual needs and preferences, and to be flexible and adaptable to your circumstances and goals. It is not a one-size-fits-all solution, but a personalized and customized plan that works for you. The new menopause diet is not about counting calories, carbs, or points, or following strict rules and restrictions.

It is not about depriving yourself of the foods you love, or feeling guilty or ashamed of your choices. It's not about going hungry or overindulging in junk food. It is not about being perfect, or never making mistakes. The new menopause diet is about eating healthy, balanced, and varied foods that nourish your body and mind, and that support your hormonal balance and health. It is about enjoying delicious food and satisfying your appetite, without feeling hungry or craving. It is about listening to your body and your intuition, and finding what works best for you. It is about being kind and compassionate to yourself, and celebrating your achievements.

The new menopause diet is not only about food, but also about other aspects of your lifestyle, such as physical activity, stress management, sleep hygiene, and social support. These factors can also affect your hormonal changes and your quality of life, and they can also be influenced by your nutrition and diet. The new menopause diet helps you integrate these factors into your daily routine, and create a holistic and harmonious approach to your health and well-being.

Furthermore, this is not a temporary or short-term fix, but a long-term and sustainable change. It is not a fad or a trend, but a lifestyle and a philosophy.

It is not a challenge or a struggle, but a joy and a pleasure. It is not a burden or a chore, but a gift and a blessing.

The new menopause diet is the ultimate guide to delicious recipes and easy hormonal change. It is the best friend you need during menopause, and beyond. It is the key to your health and happiness, and to your transformation and empowerment.

Are you ready to discover the secrets of the new menopause diet, and how to create tasty recipes that support your hormones and improve your health? Are you ready to eat well and feel great during menopause, and beyond?

If you are, then let's get started. In this chapter, we will explain the key components and features of the new menopause diet, such as the types of foods, the portions, the timing, the combinations, etc. We will also provide a list of foods to eat and foods to avoid on the new menopause diet, along with the reasons and benefits. Let's go.

# Essentials of the New Menopause Diet

The new menopause diet is based on four key components and features, which are:

- High protein: Protein is essential for your health and well-being, especially during menopause. Protein helps you feel full and satisfied, and prevents muscle loss and sarcopenia. Protein also helps you maintain or build your bone mass and strength, and prevents osteoporosis. Protein also helps you regulate your blood sugar and insulin levels, and prevents diabetes. Protein also helps you boost your metabolism and burn more calories, and prevents weight gain and obesity. Protein also helps you improve your mood and cognition, and prevents depression and dementia. Protein also helps you support your immune system and inflammation, and prevents infections and autoimmune diseases. Protein also helps you enhance your sexual function and desire, and prevents discomfort, pain, or infections. As you can see, protein is a super food for menopause, and you should include it in every meal and snack.

Aim for at least 0.8 grams of protein per kilogram of body weight per day, and choose lean and high-quality sources, such as fish, poultry, eggs, dairy, beans, nuts, and seeds.

- Low carbs: Carbs are not bad for you, but you need to be careful about the type and amount of carbs you eat, especially during menopause. Carbs can affect your hormone levels and your symptoms, and can also affect your health and well-being. Carbs can increase your blood sugar and insulin levels, and contribute to weight gain and diabetes. Carbs can also increase your inflammation and pain, and contribute to heart disease and stroke. Carbs can also affect your mood and cognition, and contribute to depression and dementia. Carbs can also affect your sleep quality and energy levels, and contribute to insomnia and fatigue. Carbs can also affect your sexual function and desire, and contribute to discomfort, pain, or infections. As you can see, carbs can be a problem for menopause, and you should limit them in your diet. Aim for no more than 20 grams of net carbs (total carbs minus fiber) per day,

And choose complex and high-fiber sources, such as fruits, vegetables, and whole grains.

- Healthy fats: Fats are not evil for you, but you need to be smart about the type and amount of fats you eat, especially during menopause. Fats can affect your hormone levels and your symptoms, and can also affect your health and well-being. Fats can lower your cholesterol, blood pressure, and inflammation, and prevent heart disease and stroke. Fats can also improve your mood, cognition, and skin health, and prevent depression, dementia, and wrinkles. Fats can also enhance your sexual function and desire, and prevent discomfort, pain, or infections. Fats can also provide you with energy and satisfaction, and prevent hunger and cravings. As you can see, fats can be a friend for menopause, and you should include them in your diet.

  Aim for at least two portions of oily fish per week, and use olive oil for cooking and dressing. Choose healthy fats that are high in omega-3 fatty acids, such as oily fish, flaxseeds, chia seeds, walnuts, and olive oil.

Avoid unhealthy fats that are high in saturated or trans fats, such as butter, cheese, cream, lard, margarine, and processed foods.

- Phytoestrogens: Phytoestrogens are plant compounds that have a similar structure and effect to estrogen. They can help balance your hormones and reduce some of the symptoms of menopause, such as hot flashes, night sweats, and vaginal dryness. They can also help prevent or manage some of the health risks and complications associated with menopause, such as osteoporosis, heart disease, stroke, diabetes, and cancer. They can also help improve your mood, cognition, and sexual function, and prevent depression, dementia, and discomfort. As you can see, phytoestrogens can be a helper for menopause, and you should include them in your diet. They can be found in foods such as soy, flaxseeds, lentils, chickpeas, and red clover, or in supplements such as isoflavones, lignans, or black cohosh. However, the safety and efficacy of phytoestrogens are not well established, and they may interact with some medications or health conditions, so consult your doctor before taking them.

These are the four key components and features of the new menopause diet, which are designed to suit your individual needs and preferences, and to be flexible and adaptable to your circumstances and goals. You can adjust the amounts and proportions of these components and features according to your symptoms, health, and well-being, and to your taste, budget, and availability. You can also experiment and find what works best for you, and what makes you feel good and happy.

In the next section, we will provide you with a list of foods to eat and foods to avoid on the new menopause diet, along with the reasons and benefits. This list is not exhaustive or definitive, but it is a good starting point and a useful reference for your diet. Let's see.

# Menopause Diet: Inclusions and Exclusions

Here is a list of foods to eat and foods to avoid on the new menopause diet, along with the reasons and benefits. This list is based on the four key components and features of the new menopause diet, which are high protein, low carb, healthy fats, and phytoestrogens. This list is not meant to be restrictive or prescriptive, but to be informative and suggestive. You can use this list as a guide, but you can also make your own choices and decisions, based on your needs and preferences, and on your symptoms, health, and well-being.

**Foods to eat:**

- Fish: Fish is a great source of protein, which helps you feel full and satisfied, and prevents muscle loss and sarcopenia. Fish is also a great source of omega-3 fatty acids, which help lower your cholesterol, blood pressure, and inflammation, and prevent heart disease and stroke. Fish also helps improve your mood, cognition, and skin health, and prevent depression, dementia, and wrinkles.

Fish also helps enhance your sexual function and desire, and prevent discomfort, pain, or infections.

Fish also provides you with energy and satisfaction, and prevents hunger and cravings. Aim for at least two portions of oily fish per week, and choose from a variety of types, such as salmon, tuna, mackerel, sardines, herring, and trout. Steer clear of mercury-rich seafood including shark, swordfish, king mackerel, and tilefish.

- Poultry: Poultry is another great source of protein, which helps you feel full and satisfied, and prevents muscle loss and sarcopenia. Poultry also helps you maintain or build your bone mass and strength, and prevents osteoporosis. Poultry also helps you regulate your blood sugar and insulin levels, and prevents diabetes. Poultry also helps you boost your metabolism and burn more calories, and prevents weight gain and obesity. Poultry also helps you improve your mood and cognition, and prevents depression and dementia.

Poultry also helps you support your immune system and inflammation, and prevents infections and autoimmune diseases. Poultry also helps you enhance your sexual function and desire, and prevent discomfort, pain, or infections. Poultry also provides you with energy and satisfaction, and prevents hunger and cravings. Aim for at least two portions of lean poultry per week, and choose from a variety of types, such as chicken, turkey, duck, and quail. Avoid poultry that is high in fat, such as skin, wings, and thighs.

- Eggs: Eggs are an excellent source of protein, which helps you feel full and satisfied, and prevents muscle loss and sarcopenia. Eggs are also an excellent source of choline, which helps improve your memory, concentration, learning, and problem-solving. Eggs also help you maintain or build your bone mass and strength, and prevent osteoporosis. Eggs also help you regulate your blood sugar and insulin levels, and prevent diabetes. Eggs also help you boost your metabolism and burn more calories, and prevent weight gain and obesity.

Eggs also help you improve your mood and cognition, and prevent depression and dementia. Eggs also help you support your immune system and inflammation, and prevent infections and autoimmune diseases.

Eggs also help you enhance your sexual function and desire, and prevent discomfort, pain, or infections. Eggs also provide you with energy and satisfaction, and prevent hunger and cravings. Aim for at least four eggs per week, and choose from a variety of ways to cook them, such as boiled, scrambled, poached, or omelet. Avoid eggs that are fried, or that have added salt, sugar, or fat.

- Dairy: Dairy is a good source of protein, which helps you feel full and satisfied, and prevents muscle loss and sarcopenia. Dairy is also a good source of calcium and vitamin D, which are essential for your bone health and prevention of osteoporosis. Dairy also helps you regulate your blood pressure and cholesterol levels, and prevent heart disease and stroke. Dairy also helps you improve your mood and cognition, and prevent depression and dementia.

Dairy also helps you support your immune system and inflammation, and prevent infections and allergies. Dairy also helps you enhance your sexual function and desire, and prevent discomfort, pain, or infections. Dairy also provides you with energy and satisfaction, and prevents hunger and cravings.

Aim for at least three portions of low-fat dairy per day, and choose from a variety of types, such as milk, yogurt, cheese, and cottage cheese. Avoid dairy that is high in fat, such as cream, butter, and ice cream.

**Some Foods to Avoid:**

- Processed foods: Processed foods are foods that have been altered from their natural state, and often contain added salt, sugar, fat, preservatives, and artificial ingredients. Processed foods can increase your blood pressure, blood sugar, cholesterol, inflammation, and weight, and can also worsen your menopausal symptoms, such as hot flashes, mood swings, insomnia, and vaginal dryness. Processed foods include candy, potato chips, fried foods, soda, energy drinks, baked goods, and ready meals.

Avoid or limit these foods as much as possible, and choose fresh, whole, and natural foods instead.

- Refined carbohydrates: Refined carbohydrates are carbs that have been stripped of their fiber, vitamins, minerals, and phytochemicals, and are quickly digested and absorbed by your body. Refined carbohydrates can spike your blood sugar and insulin levels, and contribute to weight gain, diabetes, and metabolic syndrome. Refined carbohydrates can also increase your inflammation and pain, and contribute to heart disease and stroke. Refined carbohydrates can also affect your mood and cognition, and contribute to depression and dementia. Refined carbohydrates can also affect your sleep quality and energy levels, and contribute to insomnia and fatigue. Refined carbohydrates can also affect your sexual function and desire, and contribute to discomfort, pain, or infections. Refined carbohydrates include white bread, white rice, white pasta, white flour, and white sugar. Avoid or limit these foods as much as possible, and choose complex and high-fiber carbs instead, such as fruits, vegetables, and whole grains.

- Alcohol: Alcohol is a substance that can affect your brain and body in various ways, and can have negative effects on your health and well-being, especially during menopause. Alcohol can interfere with your sleep quality, mood, and cognition, and contribute to insomnia, depression, anxiety,

  and memory loss. Alcohol can also increase your blood pressure, cholesterol, and inflammation, and increase your risk of breast cancer and osteoporosis. Alcohol can also affect your liver and kidney function, and increase your risk of liver disease and kidney stones. Alcohol can also affect your sexual function and desire, and contribute to discomfort, pain, or infections. Alcohol can also provide you with empty calories, and contribute to weight gain and obesity. Avoid or limit alcohol as much as possible, and choose water, tea, or juice instead. Aim for no more than 14 units of alcohol per week, and avoid binge drinking. One unit of alcohol is equivalent to 10 milliliters of pure alcohol, which is about half a pint of beer, a small glass of wine, or a single shot of spirits.

# Weekly Meal Plan & Shopping List

To help you get started on the new menopause diet, we have created a sample meal plan and shopping list for a week. This meal plan is based on the four key components and features of the new menopause diet, which are high protein, low carb, healthy fats, and phytoestrogens. This meal plan is also designed to be flexible and adaptable, so you can adjust it according to your needs and preferences, and to your symptoms, health, and well-being.

The meal plan provides three meals and two snacks per day, and each meal contains about 20 to 30 grams of protein, and less than 20 grams of net carbs. The snacks are optional, and you can have them whenever you feel hungry or need a boost of energy. The meal plan also includes plenty of fruits, vegetables, dairy, and phytoestrogens, to provide you with the essential vitamins, minerals, antioxidants, and phytochemicals you need for your health and well-being.

The shopping list contains all the ingredients you need to prepare the meals and snacks for the week, and it is organized by food categories, such as produce, dairy, meat, etc. The shopping list also indicates the approximate amounts and servings of each ingredient, but you can modify them according to your taste, budget, and availability. The shopping list also includes some pantry staples, such as olive oil, salt, pepper, spices, etc., that you may already have at home, but you can check and replenish them as needed.

Here is the sample meal plan and shopping list for a week:

**Day 1**

Breakfast: Greek yogurt with berries and walnuts.

Snack: Hard-boiled egg and baby carrots.

Lunch: Tuna salad with lettuce, tomatoes, cucumbers, olives, and feta cheese.

Snack: Celery sticks with peanut butter.

Dinner: Grilled chicken breast with roasted broccoli and cauliflower.

**Day 2**

Breakfast: Scrambled eggs with spinach and cheese.

Snack: Apple slices with almond butter.

Lunch: Chicken and vegetable soup with whole wheat bread.

Snack: Cottage cheese with flaxseeds and cinnamon.

Dinner: Salmon with potatoes and corn salad.

**Day 3**

Breakfast: Oatmeal with milk, chia seeds, and blueberries.

Snack: Greek yogurt with granola and dried cranberries.

Lunch: Turkey and cheese sandwich with lettuce, tomato, and mustard.

Snack: Hummus with whole wheat pita bread and cucumber slices.

Dinner: Spaghetti squash with meatballs and marinara sauce.

**Day 4**

Breakfast: Smoothie with banana, spinach, almond milk, and protein powder.

Snack: Cheese stick and grapes.

Lunch: Vegetable and bean chili with cheese and sour cream.

Snack: Edamame with sea salt.

Dinner: Steak with green beans and mushrooms.

**Day 5**

Breakfast: French toast with strawberries and whipped cream.

Snack: Trail mix with nuts, seeds, and dark chocolate.

Lunch: Chicken and avocado wrap with lettuce, tomato, and mayo.

Snack: Popcorn with parmesan cheese and garlic powder.

Dinner: Roasted pork loin with roasted Brussels sprouts and sweet potatoes.

**Day 6**

Breakfast: Pancakes with peanut butter and maple syrup.

Snack: Orange and almonds.

Lunch: Lentil and vegetable curry with brown rice.

Snack: Rice cake with cream cheese and jam.

Dinner: Baked cod with lemon and herbs, with quinoa and asparagus.

**Day 7**

Breakfast: Egg and cheese muffin with ham and spinach.

Snack: Kiwi and cashews.

Lunch: Salad with kale, quinoa, chickpeas, cherry tomatoes, and feta cheese.

Snack: Chocolate pudding with whipped cream and raspberries.

Dinner: Stir-fried tofu and vegetables with soy sauce and sesame seeds, with noodles.

## Shopping list

Produce:
- Berries (fresh or frozen): 2 cups.
- Baby carrots: 1 bag.
- Lettuce: 1 head or bag.
- Tomatoes: 4 medium.
- Cucumbers: 2 medium.
- Olives: 1/4 cup.
- Broccoli: 1 head.
- Cauliflower: 1 head.
- Spinach: 2 cups.
- Apple: 1 medium.
- Celery: 1 bunch.
- Potatoes: 4 medium.
- Corn: 2 ears or 1 can.
- Onion: 1 medium.
- Garlic: 4 cloves.
- Chia seeds: 2 tablespoons.
- Blueberries: 1/2 cup.
- Bread: 4 slices.
- Flaxseeds: 2 tablespoons.
- Cinnamon: 1 teaspoon.
- Spaghetti squash: 1 medium.
- Banana: 1 medium.

- Grapes: 1 cup.
- Cheese: 1/4 cup.
- Sour cream: 2 tablespoons.
- Green beans: 2 cups.
- Mushrooms: 1 cup.
- Strawberries: 1 cup.
- Whipped cream: 1/4 cup.
- Dried cranberries: 2 tablespoons.
- Granola: 1/4 cup.
- Mustard: 1 tablespoon.
- Hummus: 1/4 cup.
- Pita bread: 2 pieces.
- Marinara sauce: 1 cup.
- Brussels sprouts: 2 cups.
- Sweet potatoes: 2 medium.
- Dark chocolate: 1/4 cup.
- Avocado: 1 medium.
- Cheese stick: 1 piece.
- Edamame: 1 cup.
- Parmesan cheese: 2 tablespoons.
- Garlic powder: 1 teaspoon.
- Orange: 1 medium.
- Lentils: 1 cup.
- Curry powder: 1 tablespoon.
- Rice cake: 1 piece.
- Jam: 1 tablespoon.

- Lemon: 1 medium.
- Herbs: 2 tablespoons.
- Asparagus: 2 cups.
- Kiwi: 1 medium.
- Kale: 2 cups.
- Cherry tomatoes: 1 cup.
- Chickpeas: 1 cup.
- Chocolate pudding: 1 cup.
- Raspberries: 1/2 cup.
- Ham: 2 slices.

**Dairy:**
- Greek yogurt: 2 cups.
- Eggs: 14.
- Cheese: 2 cups.
- Milk: 2 cups.
- Cottage cheese: 1/2 cup.
- Butter: 2 tablespoons.
- Cream cheese: 2 tablespoons.

**Meat:**
- Tuna: 1 can or pouch.
- Chicken breast: 4 pieces.
- Turkey: 4 slices.
- Salmon: 2 fillets.
- Meatballs: 8 pieces.

- Steak: 2 pieces.
- Pork loin: 1 piece.
- Cod: 2 fillets.
- Tofu: 1 block.

**Pantry:**
- Walnuts: 1/4 cup.
- Peanut butter: 1/4 cup.
- Almond butter: 1/4 cup.
- Whole wheat bread: 1 loaf.
- Protein powder: 1/4 cup.
- Trail mix: 1/4 cup.
- Popcorn: 1/4 cup.
- Brown rice: 1 cup.
- Quinoa: 1 cup.
- Soy sauce: 2 tablespoons.
- Sesame seeds: 2 tablespoons.
- Noodles: 1 package.

**Pantry staples:**
- Olive oil: 1/4 cup.
- Salt: 1 teaspoon.
- Pepper: 1 teaspoon.
- Spices: 1/4 cup.

# Tips for Success

Following the new menopause diet may seem daunting or challenging at first, but it doesn't have to be. With some planning, preparation, and creativity, you can make the new menopause diet a part of your daily routine, and enjoy its benefits for your health and well-being. Here are some tips and tricks on how to follow the new menopause diet easily and effectively:

- Plan ahead: Planning your meals and snacks ahead of time can help you stay on track with the new menopause diet, and avoid temptations or cravings. You can use the sample meal plan and shopping list we provided as a guide, or you can create your own meal plan based on your preferences and goals. You can also use online tools or apps to help you plan, track, and monitor your food intake and nutrition. Planning ahead can also help you save time, money, and energy, and reduce food waste and stress.
- Stock your pantry: Stocking your pantry with the foods and ingredients you need for the new menopause diet can help you prepare your meals and snacks easily and quickly,

And avoid running out of options or resorting to unhealthy choices. You can use the shopping list we provided as a guide, or you can create your own shopping list based on your meal plan and budget. You can also stock up on some non-perishable or frozen foods, such as canned tuna, frozen vegetables, or frozen berries, for emergencies or convenience. Stocking your pantry can also help you avoid impulse buying or overeating, and improve your food quality and safety.

- Read labels: Reading labels can help you choose the best foods and avoid the worst foods for the new menopause diet. Reading labels can help you check the ingredients, nutrition facts, serving sizes, and expiration dates of the foods you buy and eat. Reading labels can help you compare different products and brands, and make informed and smart choices. Reading labels can help you avoid foods that are high in salt, sugar, fat, preservatives, and artificial ingredients, and choose foods that are high in protein, fiber, antioxidants, phytoestrogens,

And other beneficial compounds. Reading labels can help you control your portions and calories, and prevent overeating or under eating. Reading labels can help you identify any allergens or intolerances you may have, and prevent adverse reactions or complications. Reading labels can help you improve your food quality and safety, and prevent food poisoning or spoilage. Reading labels can also help you learn more about the foods you eat, and appreciate their value and benefits. Reading labels is a simple and effective way to follow the new menopause diet easily and effectively, and to improve your health and well-being.

# Chapter 3: Breakfast Recipes

## Greek Yogurt with Berries and Walnuts

Ingredients:

- 1 cup Greek yogurt
- 1/2 cup of berry mixture ( blueberries, strawberries, raspberries)
- 1/4 cup walnuts, chopped
- 1 tablespoon honey (optional)


- Instructions:
1. In a bowl, scoop Greek yogurt.
2. Add mixed berries on top.
3. Sprinkle chopped walnuts over the berries.
4. Drizzle honey for sweetness if desired.
5. Mix well and enjoy!
- Labels: Gluten-free, Vegetarian
- Prep Time: 5 minutes
- Cooking Time: no cooking required
- Serving Size: 1

# Scrambled Eggs with Spinach and Cheese

Ingredients:

- 2 eggs
- 1/2 cup fresh spinach, chopped
- 1/4 cup shredded cheese (your choice)
- Salt and pepper to taste
- 1 tablespoon olive oil

Instructions:

1. In a bowl, whisk eggs and season with salt and pepper.
2. Heat olive oil in a pan over medium heat.
3. Add chopped spinach to the pan and sauté until wilted.
4. Pour whisked eggs over the spinach.
5. Stir continuously until eggs are scrambled.
6. Sprinkle shredded cheese and mix until melted.
7. Serve hot!

- Labels: Gluten-free, Vegetarian
- Prep Time: 5 minutes
- Cooking Time: 5 minutes
- Serving Size: 1-2

# Oatmeal with Milk, Chia Seeds, and Blueberries

Ingredients:
- 1/2 cup rolled oats
- 1 cup milk (dairy or plant-based)
- 1 tablespoon chia seeds
- 1/2 cup blueberries
- 1 tablespoon maple syrup (optional)

Instructions:
1. In a saucepan, combine rolled oats and milk.
2. Cook over medium heat, stirring, until oats are tender.
3. Add chia seeds and mix well.
4. Remove from heat and let aside for one minute.
5. Top with blueberries and drizzle maple syrup if desired.
6. Enjoy your nutritious oatmeal!

- Labels: Gluten-free, Vegetarian
- Prep Time: 2 minutes
- Cooking Time: 5 minutes
- Serving Size: 1

# Smoothie with Banana, Spinach, Almond Milk, and Protein Powder

Ingredients:

- 1 ripe banana
- 1 cup fresh spinach
- 1 cup almond milk
- 1 scoop protein powder (plant-based for vegan option)


Instructions:

1. In a blender, combine banana, spinach, almond milk, and protein powder.

2. Blend until smooth and creamy.

3. Pour into a glass and enjoy your nutritious smoothie!


- Labels: Gluten-free, Dairy-free, Vegan
- Prep Time: 5 minutes
- Serving Size: 1

# French Toast with Strawberries and Whipped Cream

Ingredients:
- 2 slices whole wheat bread
- 2 eggs
- 1/4 cup milk (dairy or vegan)
- 1 teaspoon vanilla extract
- Strawberries, sliced
- Whipped cream

Instructions:
1. Whisk together the eggs, milk, and vanilla essence in a mixing dish.

2. Dip each slice of bread into the mixture, coating both sides.

3. Cook on a griddle or skillet over medium heat until golden brown on both sides.

4. Top with sliced strawberries and a dollop of whipped cream.

5. Serve warm and enjoy your indulgent French toast!

- Labels: Vegetarian
- Prep Time: 10 minutes
- Cooking Time: 5 minutes
- Serving Size: 1-2

# Pancakes with Peanut Butter and Maple Syrup

Ingredients:

- 1 cup pancake mix (gluten-free mix for gluten-free option)
- 3/4 cup water or milk (dairy or plant-based)
- 2 tablespoons peanut butter
- Maple syrup

Instructions:

1. In a bowl, mix pancake mix and water or milk until smooth.
2. Melt butter on a griddle or pan over medium heat.
3. Pour batter onto the griddle to form pancakes.
4. Cook until bubbles form on the surface, then flip and cook the other side.
5. Spread peanut butter between pancake layers.
6. Drizzle with maple syrup and enjoy your delicious pancakes!

- Labels: Vegetarian
- Prep Time: 5 minutes
- Cooking Time: 10 minutes
- Serving Size: 2-3

# Egg and Cheese Muffin with Ham and Spinach

**Ingredients:**

- 1 English muffin (whole grain or gluten-free for options)
- 1 egg
- 1 slice ham
- Handful of fresh spinach
- 1 slice cheese (cheddar or your preference)

**Instructions:**

1. Toast the English muffin.
2. In a skillet, cook the egg to your liking (fried or scrambled).
3. Layer the ham, fresh spinach, cooked egg, and cheese on the toasted muffin.
4. Assemble into a sandwich and enjoy!

- Labels: Vegetarian (remove ham for vegetarian), Option for Gluten-free
- Prep Time: 5 minutes
- Cooking Time: 5 minutes
- Serving Size: 1

# Soy Yogurt Parfait with Granola and Dried Cranberries

Ingredients:

- 1 cup soy yogurt
- 1/2 cup of granola (gluten-free optional)
- 2 tablespoons dried cranberries

Instructions:

1. In a glass or bowl, layer soy yogurt, granola, and dried cranberries.
2. Repeat layers.
3. Top with additional granola and cranberries.
4. Enjoy this delicious and nutritious parfait!

- Labels: Dairy-free, Vegan, Gluten-free
- Prep Time: 5 minutes
- Serving Size: 1

# Almond Flour Waffles with Cream Cheese and Raspberries

Ingredients:
- 1 cup almond flour
- 2 eggs
- 1/4 cup of milk (dairy or vegan)
- 1/2 teaspoon baking powder
- 2 tablespoons cream cheese
- Fresh raspberries

Instructions:
1. Preheat your waffle iron.
2. In a bowl, whisk together almond flour, eggs, milk, and baking powder.
3. Pour the batter into the waffle maker and cook until golden brown.
4. Spread cream cheese on the waffles and top with fresh raspberries.
5. Serve warm and enjoy these gluten-free waffles!

- Labels: Gluten-free, Vegetarian
- Prep Time: 10 minutes
- Cooking Time: 10 minutes
- Serving Size: 2-3

# Quinoa Porridge with Coconut Milk, Almonds, and Dates

Ingredients:

- 1/2 cup quinoa
- 1 cup coconut milk
- Handful of almonds, chopped
- 2 dates, pitted and chopped

Instructions:

1. Rinse quinoa under cold water.
2. In a saucepan, combine quinoa and coconut milk.
3. Bring to a boil, then reduce heat and simmer until quinoa is cooked.
4. Stir in chopped almonds and dates.
5. Serve warm and enjoy this nutritious quinoa porridge!

- Labels: Dairy-free, Vegan, Gluten-free
- Prep Time: 5 minutes
- Cooking Time: 15 minutes
- Serving Size: 1

# Chapter 4: Lunch Recipes

## Tuna Salad with Lettuce, Tomatoes, Cucumbers, Olives, and Feta Cheese

Ingredients:

- 1 can tuna, drained
- Mixed lettuce greens
- Cherry tomatoes, halved
- Cucumbers, sliced
- Kalamata olives
- Feta cheese, crumbled
- Dressing: olive oil and balsamic vinegar

Instructions:

1. In a large bowl, combine tuna, lettuce, tomatoes, cucumbers, olives, and feta cheese.

2. Toss gently with olive oil and balsamic vinegar.

3. Serve immediately and enjoy this refreshing tuna salad!

- Labels: Gluten-free
- Prep Time: 10 minutes
- Serving Size: 2

# Chicken and Vegetable Soup with Whole Wheat Bread

Ingredients:
- 1 cup cooked chicken, shredded
- Assorted vegetables (carrots, celery, onion)
- 4 cups chicken broth
- Salt and pepper to taste
- Whole wheat bread slices

Instructions:
1. In a pot, combine shredded chicken, vegetables, and chicken broth.
2. Season with salt and pepper.
3. Simmer until vegetables are tender.
4. Serve hot with whole wheat bread.
5. Enjoy this hearty chicken and vegetable soup!

- Labels: Dairy-free, Low-carb
- Prep Time: 15 minutes
- Cooking Time: 20 minutes
- Serving Size: 4

# Turkey and Cheese Sandwich with Lettuce, Tomato, and Mustard

Ingredients:
- Sliced turkey
- Cheese (your choice)
- Lettuce leaves
- Tomato slices
- Mustard
- Whole grain bread

Instructions:
1. Arrange turkey and cheese on whole grain bread.
2. Add lettuce, tomato, and spread mustard.
3. Top with another slice of bread to make a sandwich.
4. Slice and serve this classic turkey and cheese delight!

- Labels: Vegetarian (replace turkey with a plant-based alternative), Option for Gluten-free
- Prep Time: 5 minutes
- Serving Size: 1

# Vegetable and Bean Chili with Cheese and Sour Cream

Ingredients:
- Mixed beans (kidney, black, pinto)
- Assorted vegetables (bell peppers, onions, tomatoes)
- Chili powder and cumin for seasoning
- Shredded cheese and sour cream for topping

Instructions:

1. In a pot, combine mixed beans, vegetables, and seasoning.

2. Simmer until flavors meld.

3. Serve topped with shredded cheese and a dollop of sour cream.

4. Enjoy this hearty vegetable and bean chili!

- Labels: Vegan, Gluten-free
- Prep Time: 15 minutes
- Cooking Time: 30 minutes
- Serving Size: 4

# Chicken and Avocado Wrap with Lettuce, Tomato, and Mayo

Ingredients:

- Grilled chicken breast, sliced
- Avocado, sliced
- Lettuce leaves
- Tomato slices
- Whole wheat wrap
- Mayonnaise

Instructions:

1. Lay out the whole wheat wrap.
2. Place grilled chicken, avocado, lettuce, and tomato slices on the wrap.
3. Drizzle with mayonnaise.
4. Fold and wrap tightly.
5. Serve and enjoy this flavorful chicken and avocado wrap!

- Labels: Option for Gluten-free
- Prep Time: 10 minutes
- Serving Size: 1

# Lentil and Vegetable Curry with Brown Rice

Ingredients:
- 1 cup lentils
- Assorted veggies (bell peppers, spinach, carrots)
- Curry spices (cumin, coriander, turmeric)
- Cooked brown rice

Instructions:
1. Cook lentils according to package instructions.
2. In a pan, sauté vegetables and add curry spices.
3. Mix in cooked lentils and let simmer.
4. Serve over brown rice.
5. Enjoy this nutritious lentil and vegetable curry!

- Labels: Vegan, Gluten-free
- Prep Time: 15 minutes
- Cooking Time: 30 minutes
- Serving Size: 4

# Salad with Kale, Quinoa, Chickpeas, Cherry Tomatoes, and Feta Cheese

Ingredients:
- Kale, chopped
- Cooked quinoa
- Chickpeas, drained and rinsed
- Cherry tomatoes, halved
- Feta cheese, crumbled
- Olive oil and lemon dressing

Instructions:

1. In a large bowl, combine kale, quinoa, chickpeas, cherry tomatoes, and feta cheese.

2. Drizzle with olive oil and lemon dressing, toss gently.

3. Serve and enjoy this vibrant kale and quinoa salad!

- Labels: Vegetarian, Gluten-free
- Prep Time: 20 minutes
- Serving Size: 2

# Roasted Vegetable and Hummus Sandwich with Whole Wheat Pita Bread

Ingredients:
- Assorted roasted vegetables (zucchini, bell peppers, eggplant)
- Hummus
- Whole wheat pita bread

Instructions:
1. Spread hummus inside the whole wheat pita bread.
2. Stuff with roasted vegetables.
3. Slice and serve this tasty roasted vegetable and hummus sandwich!

- Labels: Vegan, Option for Gluten-free
- Prep Time: 15 minutes
- Cooking Time: 20 minutes (for roasting)
- Serving Size: 1

# Black Bean and Corn Quesadilla with Salsa and Sour Cream

Ingredients:

- Black beans, canned and drained
- Corn kernels
- Flour tortillas
- Shredded cheese (your choice)
- Salsa and sour cream for dipping

Instructions:

1. In a skillet, layer black beans, corn, and cheese between tortillas.

2. Cook until cheese melts and tortillas are golden.

3. Slice into wedges and serve with salsa and sour cream.

4. Enjoy these delightful black bean and corn quesadillas!

- Labels: Vegetarian, Option for Gluten-free
- Prep Time: 10 minutes
- Cooking Time: 10 minutes
- Serving Size: 2-3

# Tomato and Basil Soup with Mozzarella Cheese and Whole Wheat Crackers

Ingredients:
- Ripe tomatoes, diced
- Fresh basil leaves, chopped
- Mozzarella cheese, shredded
- Vegetable broth
- Whole wheat crackers

Instructions:

1. In a pot, combine diced tomatoes and vegetable broth.

2. Simmer until tomatoes are soft.

3. Stir in chopped basil and mozzarella cheese.

4. Serve hot with whole wheat crackers.

5. Enjoy this comforting tomato and basil soup!

- Labels: Vegetarian, Option for Gluten-free
- Prep Time: 10 minutes
- Cooking Time: 20 minutes
- Serving Size: 4

# Chapter 5: Dinner Recipes

## Grilled Chicken Breast with Roasted Broccoli and Cauliflower

Ingredients:
- Chicken breast: 2 pieces (about 1 pound)
- Broccoli florets: 2 cups
- Cauliflower florets: 2 cups
- Olive oil: 2 tablespoons
- Salt and pepper to taste

Instructions:
1. Preheat the grill and season chicken breasts with salt and pepper.
2. Grill chicken until fully cooked.
3. Toss broccoli and cauliflower in olive oil, salt, and pepper.
4. Roast in the oven until tender.
5. Serve grilled chicken with roasted broccoli and cauliflower.
- Labels: Gluten-free, Dairy-free, Low-carb
- Prep Time: 15 minutes
- Cooking Time: 20 minutes
- Serving Size: 2

# Salmon with Potatoes and Corn Salad

Ingredients:
- Salmon fillet: 2 pieces (about 1.5 pounds)
- Potatoes, sliced: 2 cups
- Corn kernels: 1 cup
- Olive oil: 2 tablespoons
- Lemon juice: 1 tablespoon

Instructions:
1. Preheat the oven and season salmon with olive oil, salt, and pepper.
2. Bake until fully cooked.
3. Boil or roast sliced potatoes until tender.
4. Mix corn kernels with potatoes, drizzle with lemon juice.
5. Serve salmon over the potato and corn salad.

- Labels: Gluten-free, Dairy-free
- Prep Time: 15 minutes
- Cooking Time: 20 minutes
- Serving Size: 2

# Spaghetti Squash with Meatballs and Marinara Sauce

Ingredients:

- Spaghetti squash: 1 medium-sized
- Meatballs (beef or plant-based): 1 pound
- Marinara sauce: 2 cups
- Olive oil: 2 tablespoons

Instructions:

1. Preheat oven and roast spaghetti squash until tender.
2. Cook meatballs as per package instructions.
3. Heat marinara sauce.
4. Scrape spaghetti squash into "noodles."
5. Top with meatballs and marinara sauce.

- Labels: Gluten-free, Dairy-free
- Prep Time: 15 minutes
- Cooking Time: 40 minutes
- Serving Size: 2

# Steak with Green Beans and Mushrooms

Ingredients:
- Steak: 2 pieces (about 1.5 pounds)
- Green beans, trimmed: 2 cups
- Mushrooms, sliced: 1 cup
- Olive oil: 2 tablespoons
- Garlic, minced: 2 cloves

Instructions:
1. Preheat grill or pan-sear steak to desired doneness.
2. Sauté green beans and mushrooms in olive oil and garlic.
3. Serve steak with the green bean and mushroom mixture.

- Labels: Gluten-free, Dairy-free
- Prep Time: 15 minutes
- Cooking Time: 20 minutes
- Serving Size: 2

# Roasted Pork Loin with Roasted Brussels Sprouts and Sweet Potatoes

Ingredients:

- Pork loin: 2 pounds
- Brussels sprouts, halved: 2 cups
- Sweet potatoes, cubed: 2 cups
- Olive oil: 3 tablespoons
- Rosemary and thyme for seasoning: 2 teaspoons each

Instructions:

1. Preheat the oven and season pork loin with rosemary and thyme.
2. Roast until fully cooked.
3. Toss Brussels sprouts and sweet potatoes in olive oil, salt, and pepper.
4. Roast until vegetables are golden and tender.
5. Serve roasted pork loin with Brussels sprouts and sweet potatoes.

- Labels: Gluten-free, Dairy-free, Low-carb
- Prep Time: 15 minutes
- Cooking Time: 45 minutes
- Serving Size: 2

# Baked Cod with Lemon and Herbs, with Quinoa and Asparagus

Ingredients:
- Cod fillets: 2 pieces (about 1 pound)
- Lemon: 1, sliced
- Fresh herbs (such as dill or parsley): 2 tablespoons, chopped
- Quinoa: 1 cup, uncooked
- Asparagus spears: 1 bunch
- Olive oil: 2 tablespoons
- Salt and pepper to taste

Instructions:
1. Preheat the oven and season cod with herbs, lemon slices, olive oil, salt, and pepper.
2. Bake until the cod is flaky.
3. Prepare the quinoa according per package directions.
4. Roast asparagus with olive oil, salt, and pepper.
5. Serve baked cod over a bed of quinoa with roasted asparagus.
- Labels: Gluten-free, Dairy-free
- Prep Time: 15 minutes
- Cooking Time: 20 minutes
- Serving Size: 2

# Stir-fried Tofu and Vegetables with Soy Sauce and Sesame Seeds, with Noodles

Ingredients:

- Firm tofu: 1 block (about 14 ounces), cubed
- Assorted vegetables (bell peppers, broccoli, carrots): 3 cups, sliced
- Soy sauce: 3 tablespoons
- Sesame seeds: 2 tablespoons
- Noodles of your choice: 8 ounces, cooked
- Olive oil: 2 tablespoons

Instructions:

1. Stir-fry tofu and vegetables in olive oil until tofu is golden.
2. Add soy sauce and sesame seeds, toss until well-coated.
3. Cook the noodles according to the package directions.
4. Serve stir-fried tofu and vegetables over noodles.
- Labels: Vegan
- Prep Time: 15 minutes
- Cooking Time: 15 minutes
- Serving Size: 2

# Chicken and Mushroom Casserole with Cheese and Cream

Ingredients:

- Chicken breasts: 2 pieces (about 1 pound), diced
- Mushrooms, sliced: 2 cups
- 1 cup shredded cheese (your preference)
- Heavy cream: 1 cup
- Olive oil: 2 tablespoons
- Garlic, minced: 2 cloves

Instructions:

1. Sauté chicken and mushrooms in olive oil until cooked.

2. Mix in garlic, heavy cream, and half of the cheese.

3. Transfer to a casserole dish, top with remaining cheese.

4. Bake until bubbly and golden.

5. Serve this creamy chicken and mushroom casserole.

- Labels: Option for Gluten-free
- Prep Time: 20 minutes
- Cooking Time: 30 minutes
- Serving Size: 4

# Lamb Chops with Mint Sauce, with Roasted Carrots and Parsnips

Ingredients:

- Lamb chops: 4 pieces (about 1.5 pounds)
- 1/2 cup of  chopped fresh mint leaves
- Carrots and parsnips, peeled and sliced: 2 cups
- Olive oil: 3 tablespoons
- Balsamic vinegar: 2 tablespoons
- Salt and pepper to taste

Instructions:

1. Season lamb chops with mint, olive oil, balsamic vinegar, salt, and pepper.

2. Roast lamb chops in the oven until desired doneness.

3. Toss carrots and parsnips in olive oil, salt, and pepper, and then roast.

4. Serve lamb chops with roasted carrots and parsnips.

- Labels: Gluten-free, Dairy-free
- Prep Time: 15 minutes
- Cooking Time: 25 minutes
- Serving Size: 2

# Vegetable and Tofu Lasagna with Cheese and Tomato Sauce

Ingredients:

- Lasagna noodles: 9 sheets, cooked
- Firm tofu: 1 block (about 14 ounces), crumbled
- Mixed vegetables (zucchini, bell peppers, spinach): 3 cups, chopped
- Tomato sauce: 2 cups
- 1 cup of shredded cheese (option of your choice)
- Olive oil: 2 tablespoons
- Italian seasoning: 1 tablespoon

Instructions:

1. Sauté Vegetables: In a skillet, sauté mixed vegetables in olive oil until tender.

2. Layering: Preheat oven to 375°F (190°C). Spread a thin layer of tomato sauce in a baking dish.    3. Place three lasagna noodles over the sauce.

4. Spread half of the crumbled tofu evenly over the noodles.

5. Add half of the sautéed vegetables on top of the tofu layer.

6. Pour a generous amount of tomato sauce over the vegetables.

7. Sprinkle a portion of shredded cheese over the sauce.

8. Repeat the layers with three more lasagna noodles, the remaining crumbled tofu, sautéed vegetables, tomato sauce, and shredded cheese.

9. Top with the final layer of three lasagna noodles, covering them with the remaining tomato sauce and shredded cheese.

10. Sprinkle Italian seasoning over the top for added flavor.

11. Baking: Cover the baking dish with foil and bake in the preheated oven for 30 minutes.

12. Remove the foil and bake for an additional 15 minutes or until the top is golden and the lasagna is bubbly.

13. Set aside for a few minutes to cool before slicing and serving the lasagna.

- Labels: Vegetarian, Option for Gluten-free
- Prep Time: 30 minutes
- Cooking Time: 45 minutes
- Serving Size: 6

# Chapter 6:  Snacks Recipes

## Hard-Boiled Egg and Baby Carrots

Ingredients:
- Hard-boiled eggs: 2
- Baby carrots: 1 cup

Instructions:
1. Peel the hard-boiled eggs and set aside.
2. Wash and prepare baby carrots.
3. Serve hard-boiled eggs with baby carrots.

- Labels: Gluten-free, Dairy-free, Low-carb
- Prep Time: 10 minutes
- Cooking Time: 10 minutes (for boiling eggs)
- Serving Size: 1

# Apple Slices with Almond Butter

Ingredients:
- Apples: 2, sliced
- Almond butter: 4 tablespoons


Instructions:
1. Wash and slice the apples.
2. On the apple, spread almond butter.
3. Arrange on a plate and serve


- Labels: Gluten-free, Dairy-free, Vegan
- Prep Time: 5 minutes
- Cooking Time: 0 minutes
- Serving Size: 1

# Cottage Cheese with Flax Seeds and Cinnamon

Ingredients:
  - Cottage cheese: 1 cup
  - Flaxseeds: 2 tablespoons
  - Cinnamon: 1 teaspoon

Instructions:
  1. Put the cottage cheese in a mixing bowl.
  2. Sprinkle flax seeds and cinnamon over cottage cheese.
  3. Mix well and serve.

  - Labels: Gluten-free, Vegetarian
  - Prep Time: 5 minutes
  - Cooking Time: 0 minutes
  - Serving Size: 1

# Celery Sticks with Peanut Butter

Ingredients:

- Celery sticks: 4
- Peanut butter: 4 tablespoons


Instructions:

1. Wash and cut celery sticks into manageable lengths.

2. Spread peanut butter on celery sticks.

3. Arrange on a plate and serve.


- Labels: Gluten-free, Dairy-free, Vegan
- Prep Time: 5 minutes
- Cooking Time: 0 minutes
- Serving Size: 1

# Cheese Stick and Grapes

Ingredients:
- Cheese stick: 1
- Grapes: 1 cup

Instructions:
1. Unwrap the cheese stick.
2. Wash grapes and arrange on a plate.
3. Enjoy the cheese stick with grapes.


- Labels: Gluten-free, Vegetarian
- Prep Time: 5 minutes
- Cooking Time: 0 minutes
- Serving Size: 1

# Trail Mix with Nuts, Seeds, and Dark Chocolate

Ingredients:
- Almonds: 1 cup
- Walnuts: 1/2 cup
- Pumpkin seeds: 1/4 cup
- Sunflower seeds: 1/4 cup
- Dark chocolate chunks: 1/2 cup

Instructions:
1. Mix almonds, walnuts, pumpkin seeds, sunflower seeds, and dark chocolate chunks in a bowl.
2. Toss until well combined.
3. Divide into individual servings.

- Labels: Gluten-free, Dairy-free, Vegan
- Prep Time: 5 minutes
- Cooking Time: 0 minutes
- Serving Size: 1

# Popcorn with Parmesan Cheese and Garlic Powder

Ingredients:
- Popcorn kernels: 1/2 cup (popped)
- Parmesan cheese: 2 tablespoons, grated
- Garlic powder: 1 teaspoon

Instructions:
1. Pop the popcorn kernels.
2. Sprinkle grated Parmesan cheese and garlic powder over the popcorn.
3. Toss to coat evenly.

- Labels: Gluten-free, Vegetarian
- Prep Time: 5 minutes
- Cooking Time: 5 minutes
- Serving Size: 1

# Orange and Almonds

Ingredients:
- Oranges: 2, peeled and segmented
- Almonds: 1/2 cup


Instructions:
1. Peel and segment the oranges.
2. Arrange orange segments on a plate.
3. Sprinkle almonds over the oranges.


- Labels: Gluten-free, Dairy-free, Vegan
- Prep Time: 5 minutes
- Cooking Time: 0 minutes
- Serving Size: 1

# Rice Cake with Cream Cheese and Jam

Ingredients:
- Rice cakes: 2
- Cream cheese: 4 tablespoons
- Jam (flavor of your choice): 4 tablespoons

Instructions:
1. Spread cream cheese evenly on rice cakes.
2. Add a layer of jam on top of the cream cheese.
3. Serve rice cakes with cream cheese and jam.

- Labels: Gluten-free, Vegetarian
- Prep Time: 5 minutes
- Cooking Time: 0 minutes
- Serving Size: 1

# Edamame with Sea Salt

Ingredients:

- Edamame: 1 cup, steamed
- Sea salt: 1 teaspoon

Instructions:

1. Steam the edamame until tender.
2. Sprinkle it with sea salt and toss to coat.
3. Serve edamame with sea salt.

- Labels: Gluten-free, Dairy-free, Vegan
- Prep Time: 10 minutes
- Cooking Time: 5 minutes
- Serving Size: 1

# Chapter 7: Dessert Recipes

## Chocolate Pudding with Whipped Cream and Raspberries

Ingredients:

- Chocolate pudding mix: 1 box
- Whipped cream: 1 cup
- Raspberries: 1/2 cup

Instructions:

1. Prepare chocolate pudding according to package instructions.

2. Allow the pudding to set in the refrigerator.

3. Top with a dollop of whipped cream and fresh raspberries before serving.

- Labels: Vegetarian
- Prep Time: 10 minutes
- Cooking Time: Varies (depending on pudding mix)
- Serving Size: 4

# Almond and Coconut Cookies with Dark Chocolate Chips

Ingredients:
- Almond flour: 2 cups
- Shredded coconut: 1/2 cup
- Dark chocolate chips: 1 cup
- Butter or coconut oil: 1/2 cup, melted
- Maple syrup: 1/2 cup

Instructions:
1. Preheat the oven and line a baking sheet.
2. In a bowl, mix almond flour, shredded coconut, dark chocolate chips, melted butter or coconut oil, and maple syrup.
3. Scoop cookie dough onto the baking sheet.
4. Bake until golden brown.

- Labels: Gluten-free, Vegetarian
- Prep Time: 15 minutes
- Cooking Time: 12 minutes
- Serving Size: 12 cookies

# Lemon and Blueberry Cheesecake with Almond Crust

Ingredients:
- Almond flour: 1 cup
- Cream cheese: 16 oz
- Blueberries: 1 cup
- Lemon juice: 1/4 cup
- Sugar or sweetener of choice: 1/2 cup

Instructions:

1. Preheat the oven and prepare an almond crust in a springform pan.

2. In a bowl, blend cream cheese, lemon juice, and sweetener until smooth.

3. Fold in blueberries and pour the mixture over the crust.

4. Bake until set.

- Labels: Gluten-free, Vegetarian
- Prep Time: 20 minutes
- Cooking Time: 40 minutes
- Serving Size: 8

# Peanut Butter and Banana Ice Cream with Chocolate Sauce

**Ingredients:**

- Bananas: 4, sliced and frozen
- Peanut butter: 1/2 cup
- Dark chocolate sauce: 1/4 cup

**Instructions:**

1. Blend the frozen banana slices until it turns creamy.

2. Add peanut butter and continue blending.

3. Drizzle with dark chocolate sauce before serving.

- Labels: Gluten-free, Dairy-free, Vegan
- Prep Time: 10 minutes
- Cooking Time: 0 minutes
- Serving Size: 4

# Carrot Cake with Cream Cheese Frosting

Ingredients:
- Carrots: 2 cups, grated
- Flour: 2 cups
- Sugar: 1 cup
- Eggs: 4
- Baking powder: 1 teaspoon
- Cream cheese frosting: 1 cup

Instructions:
1. Preheat the oven and prepare a carrot cake batter.
2. Bake until a toothpick inserted into the center comes out clean.
3. Allow to cool and frost with cream cheese frosting.

- Labels: Vegetarian
- Prep Time: 20 minutes
- Cooking Time: 30 minutes
- Serving Size: 10 slices

# Strawberry and Rhubarb Crumble with Oat Topping

Ingredients:
- Strawberries: 2 cups, sliced
- Rhubarb: 1 cup, chopped
- Sugar: 1/2 cup
- Flour: 2 tablespoons
- Oats: 1 cup
- Butter: 1/2 cup, melted

Instructions:
1. Preheat the oven and mix strawberries, rhubarb, sugar, and flour in a baking dish.
2. In a separate bowl, combine oats and melted butter to create the crumble topping.
3. Sprinkle the oat topping over the fruit mixture.
4. Bake until the topping is golden and the fruit is bubbly.

- Labels: Vegetarian
- Prep Time: 15 minutes
- Cooking Time: 40 minutes
- Serving Size: 6

# Chocolate and Avocado Mousse with Whipped Cream

Ingredients:
- Avocados: 2, ripe
- Cocoa powder: 1/2 cup
- Maple syrup: 1/4 cup
- Vanilla extract: 1 teaspoon
- Whipped cream: for topping

Instructions:

1. Blend avocados, cocoa powder, maple syrup, and vanilla extract until smooth.

2. Chill the mousse in the refrigerator.

3. Before serving, top with whipped cream.
- Labels: Gluten-free, Vegetarian
- Prep Time: 10 minutes
- Cooking Time: 0 minutes
- Serving Size: 4

# Apple and Cinnamon Muffins with Walnuts

Ingredients:

- Apples: 2, peeled and diced
- Flour: 2 cups
- Sugar: 1 cup
- Cinnamon: 1 teaspoon
- Walnuts: 1/2 cup, chopped
- Eggs: 2

Instructions:

1. Preheat the oven and mix apples, flour, sugar, cinnamon, walnuts, and eggs in a bowl.
2. Divide the batter among the muffin cups.
3. Bake until a toothpick comes out clean.

- Labels: Vegetarian
- Prep Time: 15 minutes
- Cooking Time: 25 minutes
- Serving Size: 12

# Pumpkin Pie with Whipped Cream

Ingredients:
- Pumpkin puree: 2 cups
- Pie crust: 1, pre-made or homemade
- Sugar: 3/4 cup
- Cinnamon: 1 teaspoon
- Whipped cream: for topping

Instructions:

1. Preheat the oven and combine pumpkin puree, sugar, and cinnamon.

2. Spoon the filling into the pie shell.

3. Bake until the middle is completely set.

4. Allow to cool and top with whipped cream before serving.

- Labels: Vegetarian
- Prep Time: 20 minutes
- Cooking Time: 50 minutes
- Serving Size: 8

# Brownies with Flaxseeds and Walnuts

Ingredients:

- Brownie mix: 1 box
- Flaxseeds: 1/4 cup
- Walnuts: 1/2 cup, chopped
- Eggs: as per brownie mix instructions

Instructions:

1. Preheat the oven and prepare brownie batter according to the mix instructions.

2. Fold in flaxseeds and chopped walnuts.

3. Bake until a toothpick comes out with fudgy crumbs.

- Labels: Vegetarian
- Prep Time: 10 minutes
- Cooking Time: Varies (according to brownie mix)
- Serving Size: 9

# Chapter 8: Soup Recipes

## Chicken and Vegetable Soup with Whole Wheat Bread

Ingredients:

- Chicken breast: 1 lb, cooked and shredded
- Mixed vegetables (carrots, celery, peas): 2 cups, chopped
- Chicken broth: 6 cups
- Whole wheat bread: 4 slices

Instructions:

1. In a pot, combine shredded chicken, mixed vegetables, and chicken broth.
2. Simmer until vegetables are tender.
3. Toast whole wheat bread and serve with the soup.

- Labels: Low-carb option available
- Prep Time: 15 minutes
- Cooking Time: 30 minutes
- Serving Size: 4

# Tomato and Basil Soup with Mozzarella Cheese and Whole Wheat Crackers

Ingredients:

- Tomatoes: 6, diced
- Fresh basil: 1/2 cup, chopped
- Mozzarella cheese: 1 cup, shredded
- Whole wheat crackers: 1 cup

Instructions:

1. In a pot, simmer diced tomatoes and fresh basil.
2. Blend the soup until smooth.
3. Serve topped with shredded mozzarella and whole wheat crackers.

- Labels: Vegetarian
- Prep Time: 20 minutes
- Cooking Time: 25 minutes
- Serving Size: 4

# Vegetable and Bean Chili with Cheese and Sour Cream

Ingredients:

- Mixed beans: 2 cans, drained and rinsed
- Mixed vegetables (bell peppers, corn, onions): 2 cups, chopped
- Tomato sauce: 2 cups
- Cheese: 1 cup, shredded
- Sour cream: for topping

Instructions:

1. In a pot, combine mixed beans, mixed vegetables, and tomato sauce.
2. Simmer until vegetables are tender.
3. Serve topped with shredded cheese and a dollop of sour cream.

- Labels: Vegetarian
- Prep Time: 15 minutes
- Cooking Time: 30 minutes
- Serving Size: 6

# Lentil and Vegetable Curry with Brown Rice

**Ingredients:**

- Lentils: 1 cup, dried
- Mixed vegetables (spinach, carrots, peas): 2 cups, chopped
- Curry sauce: 2 cups
- Brown rice: 2 cups, cooked

**Instructions:**

1. Cook lentils according to package instructions.
2. In a pan, combine cooked lentils, mixed vegetables, and curry sauce.
3. Simmer until vegetables are tender.
4. Serve over cooked brown rice.

- Labels: Vegan
- Prep Time: 20 minutes
- Cooking Time: 40 minutes
- Serving Size: 4

# Broccoli and Cheese Soup with Whole Wheat Croutons

Ingredients:
- Broccoli: 2 cups, chopped
- Cheddar cheese: 1 cup, shredded
- 4 cups of chicken or vegetable broth
- Whole wheat croutons: for topping

Instructions:
1. In a pot, combine chopped broccoli and broth.
2. Simmer until broccoli is tender.
3. Blend the soup until smooth, then stir in shredded cheddar.
4. Serve with whole wheat croutons on top.

- Labels: Vegetarian
- Prep Time: 15 minutes
- Cooking Time: 25 minutes
- Serving Size: 4

# Butternut Squash and Ginger Soup with Yogurt and Pumpkin Seeds

Ingredients:

- 1 peeled and chopped butternut squash
- Ginger: 1 tablespoon, grated
- Yogurt: 1/2 cup
- Pumpkin seeds: 2 tablespoons

Instructions:

1. In a pot, combine diced butternut squash, grated ginger, and enough water to cover.

2. Simmer until squash is tender, then blend until smooth.

3. Serve with a dollop of yogurt and a sprinkle of pumpkin seeds.

- Labels: Gluten-free, Vegetarian
- Prep Time: 15 minutes
- Cooking Time: 25 minutes
- Serving Size: 4

# Mushroom and Barley Soup with Parsley and Lemon

Ingredients:

- Mushrooms: 2 cups, sliced
- Barley: 1/2 cup, uncooked
- Parsley: 1/4 cup, chopped
- Lemon juice: 2 tablespoons

Instructions:

1. In a pot, combine sliced mushrooms, uncooked barley, and enough water to cover.

2. Simmer until the barley is tender.

3. Stir in chopped parsley and lemon juice before serving.

- Labels: Vegan
- Prep Time: 20 minutes
- Cooking Time: 40 minutes
- Serving Size: 4

# Minestrone Soup with Beans, Pasta, and Parmesan Cheese

Ingredients:
- 1 can of mixed beans (drained and rinsed)
- Pasta: 1/2 cup, uncooked
- Parmesan cheese: 1/4 cup, grated

Instructions:
1. In a pot, combine mixed beans, uncooked pasta, and enough water to cover.
2. Simmer until pasta is al dente.
3. Serve with a sprinkle of grated Parmesan cheese.

- Labels: Vegetarian
- Prep Time: 15 minutes
- Cooking Time: 20 minutes
- Serving Size: 4

# Thai Coconut and Chicken Soup with Cilantro and Lime

Ingredients:
- Chicken breast: 1, cooked and shredded
- Coconut milk: 1 can
- Cilantro: 1/4 cup, chopped
- Lime: 1, juiced

Instructions:

1. In a pot, combine shredded chicken, coconut milk, and enough water to cover.

2. Simmer until heated through.

3. Stir in chopped cilantro and lime juice before serving.

- Labels: Gluten-free
- Prep Time: 15 minutes
- Cooking Time: 20 minutes
- Serving Size: 4

# Split Pea and Ham Soup with Whole Wheat Bread

Ingredients:

- Split peas: 1 cup, dried
- Ham: 1 cup, diced
- Whole wheat bread: 4 slices

Instructions:

1. In a pot, combine dried split peas, diced ham, and enough water to cover.
2. Simmer until split peas are tender.
3. Serve with slices of whole wheat bread.


- Labels: Low-carb option available
- Prep Time: 20 minutes
- Cooking Time: 1 hour
- Serving Size: 4

# Chapter 9: Salad Recipes

## Tuna Salad with Lettuce, Tomatoes, Cucumbers, Olives, and Feta Cheese

Ingredients:
- Tuna: 1 can, drained
- Lettuce: 2 cups, shredded
- Tomatoes: 1 cup, diced
- Cucumbers: 1 cup, sliced
- Olives: 1/2 cup, sliced
- Feta cheese: 1/4 cup, crumbled

Instructions:

1. In a bowl, combine drained tuna, shredded lettuce, diced tomatoes, sliced cucumbers, sliced olives, and crumbled feta cheese.
2. Toss ingredients together.
3. Serve immediately.

- Labels: Low-carb option available
- Prep Time: 15 minutes
- Cooking Time: 0 minutes
- Serving Size: 2

# Corn Salad with Potatoes, Green Beans, and Hard-Boiled Eggs

Ingredients:
- Corn: 1 cup, cooked
- Potatoes: 1 cup, diced and boiled
- Green beans: 1 cup, blanched
- Hard-boiled eggs: 2, sliced

Instructions:
1. In a bowl, combine cooked corn, diced and boiled potatoes, blanched green beans, and sliced hard-boiled eggs.
2. Toss ingredients together.
3. Serve chilled.

- Labels: Vegetarian
- Prep Time: 20 minutes
- Cooking Time: 15 minutes
- Serving Size: 4

# Kale Salad with Quinoa, Chickpeas, Cherry Tomatoes, and Feta Cheese

Ingredients:

- Kale: 4 cups, chopped
- Quinoa: 1 cup, cooked
- 1 can of chickpeas (drained and rinsed)
- Cherry tomatoes: 1 cup, halved
- Feta cheese: 1/2 cup, crumbled

Instructions:

1. Massage chopped kale with a bit of olive oil until tender.
2. In a bowl, combine massaged kale, cooked quinoa, drained and rinsed chickpeas, halved cherry tomatoes, and crumbled feta cheese.
3. Toss ingredients together.
4. Serve chilled.

- Labels: Gluten-free, Vegetarian
- Prep Time: 25 minutes
- Cooking Time: 15 minutes
- Serving Size: 4

# Spinach Salad with Strawberries, Almonds, and Goat Cheese

Ingredients:

- Spinach: 4 cups
- Strawberries: 1 cup, sliced
- Almonds: 1/2 cup, sliced
- Goat cheese: 1/4 cup, crumbled

Instructions:

1. In a bowl, combine fresh spinach, sliced strawberries, sliced almonds, and crumbled goat cheese.

2. Toss ingredients together.

3. Serve with your favorite dressing.

- Labels: Vegetarian
- Prep Time: 15 minutes
- Cooking Time: 0 minutes
- Serving Size: 2

# Caesar Salad with Chicken, Romaine Lettuce, Croutons, and Parmesan Cheese

Ingredients:
- 1 grilled and sliced chicken breast
- Romaine lettuce: 4 cups, chopped
- Croutons: 1 cup
- Parmesan cheese: 1/2 cup, shaved

Instructions:

1. In a bowl, combine grilled and sliced chicken breast, chopped romaine lettuce, croutons, and shaved Parmesan cheese.

2. Toss ingredients together.

3. Serve with Caesar dressing.

- Labels: Low-carb option available
- Prep Time: 20 minutes
- Cooking Time: 15 minutes
- Serving Size: 4

# Greek Salad with Lettuce, Tomatoes, Cucumbers, Olives, and Feta Cheese

Ingredients:
- Lettuce: 4 cups, chopped
- Tomatoes: 1 cup, diced
- Cucumbers: 1 cup, sliced
- Olives: 1/2 cup, sliced
- Feta cheese: 1/2 cup, crumbled

Instructions:

1. In a large bowl, combine chopped lettuce, diced tomatoes, sliced cucumbers, sliced olives, and crumbled feta cheese.
2. Toss ingredients together.
3. Serve with Greek dressing.

- Labels: Vegetarian
- Prep Time: 15 minutes
- Cooking Time: 0 minutes
- Serving Size: 2

# Cobb Salad with Chicken, Bacon, Avocado, Eggs, and Blue Cheese

Ingredients:
- 1 grilled and sliced chicken breast
- Bacon: 6 strips, cooked and crumbled
- Avocado: 1, diced
- Eggs: 2, hard-boiled and sliced
- Blue cheese: 1/2 cup, crumbled

Instructions:

1. Arrange grilled and sliced chicken breast, crumbled bacon, diced avocado, sliced hard-boiled eggs, and crumbled blue cheese on a bed of lettuce.

2. Toss ingredients together.

3. Serve with your favorite dressing.

- Labels: Low-carb option available
- Prep Time: 25 minutes
- Cooking Time: 15 minutes
- Serving Size: 2

# Asian Salad with Cabbage, Carrots, Edamame, Peanuts, and Sesame Dressing

Ingredients:
- Cabbage: 4 cups, shredded
- Carrots: 1 cup, julienned
- Edamame: 1 cup, cooked
- Peanuts: 1/2 cup
- Sesame dressing: 1/4 cup

Instructions:
1. In a bowl, combine shredded cabbage, julienned carrots, cooked edamame, and peanuts.
2. Toss ingredients together.
3. Drizzle with sesame dressing before serving.
- Labels: Vegan
- Prep Time: 20 minutes
- Cooking Time: 5 minutes
- Serving Size: 4

# Waldorf Salad with Apples, Celery, Walnuts, and Mayonnaise

Ingredients:
- Apples: 2, diced
- Celery: 1 cup, sliced
- Walnuts: 1/2 cup, chopped
- Mayonnaise: 1/4 cup

Instructions:

1. In a bowl, combine diced apples, sliced celery, chopped walnuts, and mayonnaise.

2. Toss ingredients together.

3. Serve chilled.


- Labels: Vegetarian
- Prep Time: 15 minutes
- Cooking Time: 0 minutes
- Serving Size: 2

# Caprese Salad with Tomatoes, Mozzarella Cheese, Basil, and Balsamic Vinegar

Ingredients:
- Tomatoes: 4, sliced
- Mozzarella cheese: 1 cup, sliced
- Basil: 1/2 cup, fresh
- Balsamic vinegar: 2 tablespoons

Instructions:
1. Arrange sliced tomatoes, sliced mozzarella cheese, and fresh basil on a serving platter.
2. Drizzle with balsamic vinegar before serving.

- Labels: Gluten-free, Vegetarian
- Prep Time: 15 minutes
- Cooking Time: 0 minutes
- Serving Size: 2

# Chapter 10: Smoothies Recipes

## Smoothie with Banana, Spinach, Almond Milk, and Protein Powder

Ingredients:
- Banana: 1, ripe
- Spinach: 1 cup
- Almond milk: 1 cup
- Protein powder: 1 scoop

Instructions:

1. Blend ripe banana, spinach, almond milk, and protein powder until smooth.
2. Serve immediately and enjoy.

- Labels: Gluten-free, Vegan
  - Prep Time: 5 minutes
  - Cooking Time: 0 minutes
  - Serving Size: 1

# Smoothie with Blueberries, Yogurt, Milk, and Flaxseeds

Ingredients:
- Blueberries: 1 cup
- Yogurt: 1/2 cup
- Milk: 1 cup
- Flaxseeds: 1 tablespoon

Instructions:

1. Blend blueberries, yogurt, milk, and flaxseeds until well combined.

2. Serve immediately and enjoy
- Labels: Vegetarian
- Prep Time: 5 minutes
- Cooking Time: 0 minutes
- Serving Size: 1

# Smoothie with Mango, Pineapple, Coconut Milk, and Chia Seeds:

Ingredients:
- Mango: 1 cup, diced
- Pineapple: 1 cup, diced
- Coconut milk: 1 cup
- Chia seeds: 1 tablespoon

Instructions:

1. Blend diced mango, diced pineapple, coconut milk, and chia seeds until smooth.
2. Serve immediately and enjoy

- Labels: Vegan
- Prep Time: 5 minutes
- Cooking Time: 0 minutes
- Serving Size: 1

# Smoothie with Strawberries, Yogurt, Milk, and Granola

Ingredients:
- Strawberries: 1 cup, sliced
- Yogurt: 1/2 cup
- Milk: 1 cup
- Granola: 1/4 cup

Instructions:

1. Blend sliced strawberries, yogurt, milk, and granola until well combined.

2. Serve immediately and enjoy

- Labels: Vegetarian
- Prep Time: 5 minutes
- Cooking Time: 0 minutes
- Serving Size: 1

# Smoothie with Peanut Butter, Banana, Milk, and Cocoa Powder

Ingredients:
- Peanut butter: 2 tablespoons
- Banana: 1, ripe
- Milk: 1 cup
- Cocoa powder: 1 tablespoon

Instructions:

1. Blend peanut butter, ripe banana, milk, and cocoa powder until smooth.

2. Serve immediately and enjoy

- Labels: Vegetarian
- Prep Time: 5 minutes
- Cooking Time: 0 minutes
- Serving Size: 1

# Smoothie with Avocado, Spinach, Milk, and Honey

**Ingredients:**
- Avocado: 1/2, ripe
- Spinach: 1 cup
- Milk: 1 cup
- Honey: 1 tablespoon

**Instructions:**

1. Blend ripe avocado, spinach, milk, and honey until smooth.

2. Serve immediately and enjoy

- Labels: Vegetarian
- Prep Time: 5 minutes
- Cooking Time: 0 minutes
- Serving Size: 1

# Smoothie with Cherries, Yogurt, Milk, and Almond Extract

Ingredients:
- Cherries: 1 cup, pitted
- Yogurt: 1/2 cup
- Milk: 1 cup
- Almond extract: 1/2 teaspoon

Instructions:

1. Blend pitted cherries, yogurt, milk, and almond extract until well combined.

2. Serve immediately and enjoy

- Labels: Vegetarian
- Prep Time: 5 minutes
- Cooking Time: 0 minutes
- Serving Size: 1

# Smoothie with Peaches, Yogurt, Milk, and Vanilla Extract

Ingredients:
- Peaches: 1 cup, sliced
- Yogurt: 1/2 cup
- Milk: 1 cup
- Vanilla extract: 1/2 teaspoon

Instructions:

1. Blend sliced peaches, yogurt, milk, and vanilla extract until smooth.

2. Serve immediately and enjoy.

- Labels: Vegetarian
- Prep Time: 5 minutes
- Cooking Time: 0 minutes
- Serving Size: 1

# Smoothie with Raspberries, Yogurt, Milk, and Lemon Juice

Ingredients:

- Raspberries: 1 cup
- Yogurt: 1/2 cup
- Milk: 1 cup
- Lemon juice: 1 tablespoon

Instructions:

1. Blend raspberries, yogurt, milk, and lemon juice until well combined.

2. Serve immediately and enjoy

- Labels: Vegetarian
- Prep Time: 5 minutes
- Cooking Time: 0 minutes
- Serving Size: 1

# Smoothie with Kiwi, Spinach, Milk, and Ginger

Ingredients:
- Kiwi: 1, peeled and sliced
- Spinach: 1 cup
- Milk: 1 cup
- Ginger: 1/2 teaspoon, grated

Instructions:

1. Blend sliced kiwi, spinach, milk, and grated ginger until smooth.

2. Serve immediately and enjoy

- Labels: Vegetarian
- Prep Time: 5 minutes
- Cooking Time: 0 minutes
- Serving Size: 1

# Chapter 11: Main Courses

## Grilled Chicken Breast with Roasted Broccoli and Cauliflower

Ingredients:
- Chicken breast: 2, boneless and skinless
- Broccoli: 2 cups, florets
- Cauliflower: 2 cups, florets
- Olive oil: 2 tablespoons
- Salt and pepper to taste

Instructions:
1. Preheat the grill.
2. Season chicken breasts with salt and pepper.
3. Grill chicken until fully cooked.
4. Toss broccoli and cauliflower with olive oil, salt, and pepper.
5. Roast in the oven until tender.
6. Serve grilled chicken with roasted broccoli and cauliflower.
- Labels: Low-carb, Gluten-free
- Prep Time: 15 minutes
- Cooking Time: 25 minutes
- Serving Size: 2

# Salmon with Potatoes and Corn Salad

**Ingredients:**

- Salmon fillets: 2
- Potatoes: 4 medium, diced
- Corn: 1 cup, cooked
- Olive oil: 3 tablespoons
- Lemon juice: 2 tablespoons

**Instructions:**

1. Preheat the oven.
2. Season salmon with salt, pepper, and lemon juice.
3. Bake salmon until flaky.
4. Boil diced potatoes until tender.
5. Toss potatoes and corn with olive oil, salt, and pepper.
6. Serve salmon over the potato and corn salad.

- Labels: Gluten-free
- Prep Time: 20 minutes
- Cooking Time: 30 minutes
- Serving Size: 2

# Spaghetti Squash with Meatballs and Marinara Sauce

Ingredients:
- Spaghetti squash: 1
- Meatballs: 16, cooked
- Marinara sauce: 2 cups
- Parmesan cheese: 1/2 cup, grated

Instructions:
1. Preheat the oven.
2. Roast spaghetti squash until fork-tender.
3. Heat meatballs in marinara sauce.
4. Scrape spaghetti squash into strands.
5. Top with meatballs, marinara sauce, and Parmesan cheese.
6. Serve and enjoy.

- Labels: Low-carb, Gluten-free
- Prep Time: 15 minutes
- Cooking Time: 45 minutes
- Serving Size: 2

# Steak with Green Beans and Mushrooms:

## Ingredients:
- Steak: 2, your choice of cut
- Green beans: 2 cups, trimmed
- Mushrooms: 2 cups, sliced
- Olive oil: 2 tablespoons

## Instructions:
1. Season the steaks very well with salt and pepper.
2. Cook steaks to desired doneness.
3. Sauté green beans and mushrooms in olive oil until tender.
4. Serve steaks with green beans and mushrooms.

- Labels: Gluten-free
- Prep Time: 15 minutes
- Cooking Time: 20 minutes
- Serving Size: 2

# Roasted Pork Loin with Roasted Brussels Sprouts and Sweet Potatoes

Ingredients:
- Pork loin: 1 pound
- Brussels sprouts: 2 cups, halved
- Sweet potatoes: 2 cups, diced
- Olive oil: 3 tablespoons
- Rosemary: 1 teaspoon, dried

Instructions:
1. Preheat the oven.
2. Rub pork loin with olive oil and dried rosemary.
3. Roast pork loin until cooked.
4. Toss Brussels sprouts and sweet potatoes in olive oil, salt, and pepper.
5. Roast vegetables until golden.
6. Serve sliced pork loin with roasted Brussels sprouts and sweet potatoes.

- Labels: Gluten-free
- Prep Time: 20 minutes
- Cooking Time: 45 minutes
- Serving Size: 2

# Baked Cod with Lemon and Herbs, with Quinoa and Asparagus

Ingredients:

- Cod fillets: 2
- Lemon: 1, sliced
- Fresh herbs (rosemary, thyme): 2 tablespoons, chopped
- Quinoa: 1 cup, cooked
- Asparagus: 1 bunch, trimmed
- Olive oil: 3 tablespoons
- Salt and pepper to taste

Instructions:

1. Preheat the oven.
2. Place cod fillets on a baking sheet.
3. Drizzle with olive oil, lemon slices, fresh herbs, salt, and pepper.
4. Bake until the cod is flaky.
5. Serve over cooked quinoa with roasted asparagus on the side.

- Labels: Gluten-free
- Prep Time: 15 minutes
- Cooking Time: 20 minutes
- Serving Size: 2

# Stir-Fried Tofu and Vegetables with Soy Sauce and Sesame Seeds, with Noodles

Ingredients:

- Tofu: 1 block, cubed
- Mixed vegetables (broccoli, bell peppers, carrots): 2 cups, chopped
- Soy sauce: 3 tablespoons
- Sesame seeds: 1 tablespoon
- Noodles: 8 oz, cooked
- Sesame oil: 2 tablespoons

Instructions:

1. Stir-fry tofu and mixed vegetables in sesame oil.
2. Add soy sauce and sesame seeds.
3. Cook until vegetables are tender.
4. Serve over cooked noodles.

- Labels: Vegan, Vegetarian
- Prep Time: 15 minutes
- Cooking Time: 15 minutes
- Serving Size: 2

# Chicken and Mushroom Casserole with Cheese and Cream

Ingredients:

- 2 boneless and skinless chicken breasts
- Mushrooms: 2 cups, sliced
- Cheese: 1 cup, shredded
- Cream: 1/2 cup
- Garlic: 2 cloves, minced
- Thyme: 1 teaspoon, dried

Instructions:

1. Preheat the oven.
2. Season chicken breasts with salt, pepper, and dried thyme.
3. Sear chicken until browned.
4. In a casserole dish, layer chicken, mushrooms, garlic, cream, and cheese.
5. Bake until bubbly and golden.
6. Serve hot.

- Labels: Gluten-free
- Prep Time: 20 minutes
- Cooking Time: 30 minutes
- Serving Size: 2

# Lamb Chops with Mint Sauce, with Roasted Carrots and Parsnips

Ingredients:
- Lamb chops: 4
- Mint sauce: 1/4 cup
- Carrots: 1 cup, sliced
- Parsnips: 1 cup, sliced
- Olive oil: 2 tablespoons
- Rosemary: 1 teaspoon, dried

Instructions:
1. Preheat the oven.
2. Rub lamb chops with olive oil and dried rosemary.
3. Roast lamb chops until cooked.
4. Toss sliced carrots and parsnips with olive oil, salt, and pepper.
5. Roast vegetables until tender.
6. Serve lamb chops with mint sauce and roasted carrots and parsnips.

- Labels: Gluten-free
- Prep Time: 15 minutes
- Cooking Time: 30 minutes
- Serving Size: 2

# Vegetable and Tofu Lasagna with Cheese and Tomato Sauce

Ingredients:

- Lasagna noodles: 8 oz, cooked
- Tofu: 1 block, crumbled
- Mixed vegetables (zucchini, bell peppers, spinach): 2 cups, chopped
- Cheese: 1 cup, shredded
- Tomato sauce: 2 cups
- Garlic: 2 cloves, minced
- Italian seasoning: 1 teaspoon

Instructions:

1. Preheat the oven.
2. In a baking dish, layer lasagna noodles, crumbled tofu, mixed vegetables, cheese, garlic, tomato sauce, and Italian seasoning.
3. Repeat layers.
4. Bake until bubbly and golden.
5. Serve hot.

- Labels: Vegetarian
- Prep Time: 30 minutes
- Cooking Time: 45 minutes
- Serving Size: 4

# Chapter 12: Side Dishes

## Roasted Broccoli and Cauliflower

Ingredients:
- Broccoli: 2 cups, florets
- Cauliflower: 2 cups, florets
- Olive oil: 2 tablespoons
- Salt and pepper to taste

Instructions:
1. Preheat the oven.
2. Toss broccoli and cauliflower with olive oil, salt, and pepper.
3. Roast in the oven until tender and slightly crispy.
4. Serve hot.

- Labels: Gluten-free, Vegan
- Prep Time: 10 minutes
- Cooking Time: 20 minutes
- Serving Size: 2

# Potatoes and Corn Salad

Ingredients:

- Potatoes: 4 medium, diced
- Corn: 1 cup, cooked
- Olive oil: 3 tablespoons
- Lemon juice: 2 tablespoons
- Salt and pepper to taste

Instructions:

1. Boil diced potatoes until tender.
2. Toss potatoes and cooked corn with olive oil, lemon juice, salt, and pepper.
3. Serve chilled.

- Labels: Gluten-free, Vegan
- Prep Time: 15 minutes
- Cooking Time: 15 minutes
- Serving Size: 4

# Green Beans and Mushrooms

Ingredients:
- Green beans: 2 cups, trimmed
- Mushrooms: 2 cups, sliced
- Olive oil: 2 tablespoons
- Garlic: 2 cloves, minced
- Salt and pepper to taste

Instructions:
1. Sauté green beans and mushrooms in olive oil until tender.
2. Add salt, pepper and minced garlic.
3. Cook until garlic is fragrant.
4. Serve hot.
- Labels: Gluten-free, Vegan
- Prep Time: 10 minutes
- Cooking Time: 15 minutes
- Serving Size: 2

# Roasted Brussels Sprouts and Sweet Potatoes

Ingredients:
- Brussels sprouts: 2 cups, halved
- Sweet potatoes: 2 cups, diced
- Olive oil: 3 tablespoons
- Maple syrup: 2 tablespoons
- Salt and pepper to taste

Instructions:
1. Preheat the oven.
2. Toss Brussels sprouts and sweet potatoes with olive oil, maple syrup, salt, and pepper.
3. Roast until caramelized and tender.
4. Serve hot.

- Labels: Gluten-free, Vegan
- Prep Time: 15 minutes
- Cooking Time: 30 minutes
- Serving Size: 2

# Quinoa and Asparagus

Ingredients:
- Quinoa: 1 cup, cooked
- Asparagus: 1 bunch, trimmed
- Lemon zest: 1 teaspoon
- Olive oil: 2 tablespoons
- Salt and pepper to taste

Instructions:
1. Cook the quinoa the way it is directed on package
2. Steam or boil asparagus until tender.
3. Toss quinoa and asparagus with olive oil, lemon zest, salt, and pepper.
4. Serve warm.

- Labels: Gluten-free, Vegan
- Prep Time: 15 minutes
- Cooking Time: 20 minutes
- Serving Size: 2

# Noodles

**Ingredients:**
- Noodles: 8 oz.
- Water: As per package instructions
- Salt: 1 teaspoon

**Instructions:**
1. Boil water with salt.
2. Cook noodles until al dente.
3. Rinse with cold water after draining.
4. Use as desired in recipes.

- Labels: Vegan
- Prep Time: 5 minutes
- Cooking Time: 8-10 minutes
- Serving Size: Varies

# Cheese and Cream

- Ingredients:
    - Cheese: 1 cup, shredded
    - Cream: 1/2 cup

Instructions:
    1. Combine shredded cheese and cream in a bowl.
    2. Use as a topping or in recipes as specified.


- Labels: Vegetarian
- Prep Time: 2 minutes
- Cooking Time:
- Serving Size: Varies

# Roasted Carrots and Parsnips

Ingredients:
- Carrots: 1 cup, sliced
- Parsnips: 1 cup, sliced
- Olive oil: 2 tablespoons
- Salt and pepper to taste

Instructions:
1. Preheat the oven.
2. Season the carrots and parsnips with salt and pepper.
3. Roast until tender and caramelized.
4. Serve hot.

- Labels: Gluten-free, Vegan
- Prep Time: 10 minutes
- Cooking Time: 25 minutes
- Serving Size: 2

# Tomato Sauce

**Ingredients:**

- Tomatoes: 6, ripe and diced
- Olive oil: 2 tablespoons
- Garlic: 2 cloves, minced
- Basil: 1 tablespoon, fresh, chopped
- Salt and pepper to taste

**Instructions:**

1. Sauté minced garlic in olive oil until fragrant.
2. Add diced tomatoes, basil, salt, and pepper.
3. Simmer until tomatoes break down.
4. Use as a sauce in various recipes.

- Labels: Vegan
- Prep Time: 10 minutes
- Cooking Time: 20 minutes
- Serving Size: Varies

# Whole Wheat Bread

Ingredients:
- Whole wheat flour: 3 cups
- Water: 1 1/4 cups
- Yeast: 2 teaspoons
- Salt: 1 teaspoon

Instructions:

1. Combine yeast and warm water, let it sit for 5 minutes.
2. In a large bowl, mix whole wheat flour and salt.
3. Add the yeast mixture, knead until smooth.
4. Let the dough rise, then shape into a loaf.
5. Bake until golden brown.

- Labels: Vegan
- Prep Time: 20 minutes + rising time
- Cooking Time: 30 minutes
- Serving Size: Varies

# Chapter 13: The New Menopause Diet Lifestyle

Menopause is a natural change that affects each woman in a unique way. Some women may endure hot flashes, mood fluctuations, weight gain, or bone loss, while others may encounter just little discomfort. Whatever your symptoms are, you can take control of your health and well-being by eating a balanced and nutritious diet tailored to your own requirements and tastes.

In this chapter, we will discuss how the new menopause diet can help you achieve your health and wellness goals, such as losing weight, reducing inflammation, boosting energy, improving mood, and more. We will also give you some practical tips and examples of foods to eat and avoid during this time of change. By the end of this chapter, you will have a better understanding of how to nourish your body and mind during menopause and beyond.

# How the new menopause diet can help you

The new menopause diet is not a one-size-fits-all approach, but rather a flexible and personalized way of eating that takes into account your individual needs, symptoms, and preferences. It is based on the following principles:

- Eat a variety of foods from all the food groups, especially fruits, vegetables, whole grains, lean proteins, healthy fats, and calcium-rich foods.
- Avoid or limit foods that may worsen your symptoms, such as refined sugars, processed foods, alcohol, caffeine, and spicy foods.
- Include foods that may help with your symptoms, such as soy, flaxseeds, nuts, fish, and legumes, which contain phytoestrogens, omega-3 fatty acids, and other beneficial nutrients.
- Stay hydrated by drinking lots of water throughout the day.
- Adjust your calorie intake and portion sizes according to your activity level and metabolism, which may slow down during menopause.

- Enjoy your food and eat mindfully, paying attention to your hunger and fullness cues, and savoring every bite.

By following these principles, you can reap the following benefits from the new menopause diet:

- Lose weight or maintain a healthy weight. Eating a balanced diet that is rich in fiber, protein, and healthy fats can help you feel fuller for longer and prevent overeating. It can also help you burn more calories and preserve your muscle mass, which may decline during menopause. Additionally, avoiding or limiting foods that are high in calories, fat, and sugar can help you reduce your calorie intake and prevent weight gain.
- Reduce inflammation to lessen your chances of developing chronic illnesses. Eating a variety of fruits, vegetables, whole grains, nuts, seeds, and fish can provide you with antioxidants, anti-inflammatory compounds, and other phytochemicals that can help protect your cells from damage and lower your risk of diseases such as diabetes, heart disease, and cancer.

These foods can also help lower your blood pressure, cholesterol, and blood sugar levels, which may increase during menopause.

- Boost your energy and mood. Eating a balanced diet that provides you with adequate carbohydrates, protein, and healthy fats can help you maintain your blood sugar levels and prevent energy crashes and mood swings. Carbohydrates are the main source of fuel for your brain and muscles, while protein and healthy fats can help you feel satisfied and support your hormone production. Eating foods that are rich in B vitamins, iron, magnesium, and zinc can also help you combat fatigue, depression, anxiety, and irritability, which may affect you during menopause.

- Support your bone health and prevent osteoporosis. Eating foods that are rich in calcium, vitamin D, magnesium, and phosphorus can help you build and maintain strong bones, which may become weaker and more prone to fractures during menopause. Calcium and vitamin D are especially important, as they work together to help your body absorb and use calcium.

Dairy products, leafy greens, fortified cereals, and fish are good sources of calcium and vitamin D. You can also take supplements if you are not getting enough from your diet.

# Menopause Diet Success Stories

You may be wondering if the new menopause diet really works, and if it can make a difference in your life. To answer that, we have gathered some success stories and testimonials from real women who have tried and benefited from the new menopause diet. These women have shared their personal experiences, challenges, and achievements with us, and we hope they will inspire and motivate you to give the new menopause diet a try.

### Lisa's story

Lisa, 48, from Dalton, Cumbria, was suffering from severe perimenopause symptoms, such as anxiety, stress, memory loss, and confusion. She was worried she had dementia or Alzheimer's disease, and she felt overwhelmed by her work and life. She tried several GPs, but none of them could help her. She decided to pay for a private doctor, who prescribed her hormone replacement therapy (HRT).

However, HRT alone was not enough to solve her problems. She also needed to change her diet and lifestyle. She found out about the new menopause diet online, and decided to give it a go. She started to eat more fruits, vegetables, whole grains, soy, flaxseeds, nuts, fish, and legumes, and avoided or limited refined sugars, processed foods, alcohol, caffeine, and spicy foods. She also drank more water and ate mindfully. She noticed a significant improvement in her energy, mood, and mental clarity. She felt less anxious and stressed, and more confident and happy. She also lost some weight and felt more comfortable in her body.

Lisa said: "The new menopause diet has changed my life. I feel like a new person. I have more energy, more focus, and more joy. I can handle my work and life better, and I don't feel overwhelmed anymore. I also look better and feel healthier. I wish I had known about this diet sooner. It has made a huge difference in my perimenopause journey."

### Paula's story

Paula, 52, from London, was a vice-principal at a school, enjoying the challenges of teaching and management. However, when she hit menopause, she started to experience hot flashes, mood swings, weight gain, and bone loss.

She also lost her confidence and assertiveness, and felt unable to cope with her role. She decided to step back from her position, and work as a part-time teacher instead. She felt frustrated and disappointed with herself, and wondered if she could ever get back to her old self. She heard about the new menopause diet from a friend, who had tried it and recommended it to her. She decided to give it a shot, and followed the principles of eating a balanced and nutritious diet that suited her needs and preferences. She ate more calcium-rich foods, such as dairy products, leafy greens, fortified cereals, and fish, to support her bone health. She also ate more foods that contained phytoestrogens, omega-3 fatty acids, and other beneficial nutrients, such as soy, flaxseeds, nuts, fish, and legumes, to help with her symptoms. She avoided or limited foods that worsened her symptoms, such as refined sugars, processed foods, alcohol, caffeine, and spicy foods. She drank plenty of water and stayed hydrated. She also enjoyed her food and ate mindfully, paying attention to her hunger and fullness cues, and savoring every bite.

She noticed a remarkable improvement in her symptoms, especially her hot flashes, mood swings, and weight gain. She felt cooler, calmer, and lighter.

She also regained her confidence and assertiveness, and felt more in control of her health and well-being. She decided to pursue an MA in counseling, and hoped to support other women going through the same thing. Paula said: "The new menopause diet has helped me a lot. I feel better physically, mentally, and emotionally. I have less symptoms, and more self-esteem. I have also found a new purpose and passion in life. I want to help other women who are struggling with menopause, and show them that there is hope and happiness after the change."

## Tips for Long-Term Success

The new menopause diet is not a temporary fix, but a lifelong commitment to your health and well-being. It may not be easy to stick to it at first, especially if you are used to eating differently or have a busy schedule. However, with some planning, preparation, and perseverance, you can make the new menopause diet a part of your daily routine and enjoy its benefits for years to come. Here are some tips and suggestions on how to maintain and sustain the new menopause diet in the long term, as well as how to cope with potential challenges and setbacks:

- Set realistic and specific goals: Instead of aiming for a vague or unrealistic goal, such as losing a certain amount of weight or never eating a certain food again, set smaller and more achievable goals, such as eating more vegetables, reducing your portion sizes, or limiting your alcohol intake. Make a list of your goals and keep track of your progress on a regular basis. Celebrate your successes and reward yourself with something healthy and enjoyable, such as a massage, a new book, or a hobby.

- Plan ahead and prepare your meals: One of the biggest challenges of following the new menopause diet is finding the time and energy to cook healthy meals. To avoid resorting to takeaways, processed foods, or skipping meals, plan your meals ahead of time and prepare them in advance. You can use a weekly menu planner, a shopping list, and a batch cooking method to make your life easier. You can also freeze some meals for later use, or use a slow cooker, an instant pot, or a pressure cooker to save time and effort.

- Eat mindfully and enjoy your food: Eating mindfully means paying attention to your hunger and fullness cues, eating slowly and without distractions, and savoring every bite. Eating mindfully can help you eat less, digest better, and appreciate your food more. It can also help you cope with emotional eating, which is a common problem during menopause. Instead of using food as a way to cope with stress, boredom, loneliness, or sadness, find other ways to soothe yourself, such as talking to a friend, listening to music, meditating, or journaling.

- Be flexible and adaptable: The new menopause diet is not a rigid or restrictive diet, but a flexible and adaptable one. It allows you to eat a variety of foods from all the food groups, as long as they are nutritious and suit your needs and preferences. It also allows you to enjoy occasional treats, such as a piece of cake, a glass of wine, or a pizza, as long as they are not too frequent or too large. The key is to find a balance that works for you and your lifestyle, and to make adjustments as needed.

For example, if you are traveling, eating out, or celebrating a special occasion, you can choose the healthiest options available, or eat smaller portions, or compensate by eating lighter meals before or after.

- Seek support and guidance: Following the new menopause diet can be challenging, especially if you feel alone or unsupported. That's why it's important to seek support and guidance from others who are going through the same thing, or who can help you along the way. You can join a support group, an online community, or a class that focuses on menopause and nutrition. You can also talk to your doctor, a dietitian, a therapist, or a coach who can provide you with professional advice and guidance. You can also involve your family, friends, or partner in your journey, and ask them to join you, encourage you, or respect your choices.

# CONCLUSION

You have reached the end of this book, and we hope you have enjoyed reading it as much as we have enjoyed writing it. This book was written with the aim of helping you navigate the menopause transition with ease and grace, by providing you with the latest information, research, and advice on how to eat well and live well during this time of change.

In this book, you have learned about:

- What menopause is, what causes it, and what are the common symptoms and health risks associated with it
- How your diet and nutrition can affect your menopause experience, and what are the key nutrients and foods you need to include or avoid in your diet
- How the new menopause diet can help you achieve your health and wellness goals, such as losing weight, reducing inflammation, boosting energy, improving mood, and more
- How to follow the new menopause diet principles, and what are some practical tips and examples of foods to eat and avoid during menopause.

- How to plan, prepare, and cook delicious and nutritious meals that suit your needs and preferences, and what are some easy and tasty recipes you can try at home
- How to maintain and sustain the new menopause diet in the long term, and how to cope with potential challenges and setbacks
- How other women have tried and benefited from the new menopause diet, and what are their success stories and testimonials

By reading this book, you have taken a big step towards improving your health and happiness during menopause and beyond. You have gained the knowledge, skills, and confidence to make positive changes in your diet and lifestyle, and to embrace the new menopause diet as a way of living, not just a way of eating.

We congratulate and encourage you for completing this book and embarking on the new menopause diet journey. We are proud of you and we are here to support you along the way. Keep in mind that you are not alone on this endeavor. You are part of a community of women who are going through the same thing, and who are ready to share their experiences, insights, and tips with you.

We invite you to share your feedback and experiences with us and other readers. You can contact us through our website, email, or social media, and let us know what you think of this book, how the new menopause diet has helped you, and what challenges or questions you have faced or have. You can also join our online forum, where you can connect with other women who are following the new menopause diet, and exchange ideas, recipes, and stories.

We thank you for choosing this book and trusting us with your health and well-being. We hope this book has been valuable and helpful for you, and that it has inspired you to take charge of your menopause journey and make it a positive and empowering one. We wish you all the best and we look forward to hearing from you soon.